FUNCTIONAL STRENGTH TRAINING FOR PHYSICAL EDUCATION

Nate VanKouwenberg

Next Level Strength and Conditioning

Victor Central Schools

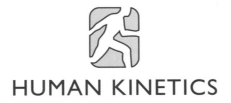

Library of Congress Cataloging-in-Publication Data

Names: VanKouwenberg, Nate, 1981- author.
Title: Functional strength training for physical education / Nate
   VanKouwenberg.
Description: Champaign, IL : Human Kinetics, 2025. | Includes
   bibliographical references.
Identifiers: LCCN 2023031845 (print) | LCCN 2023031846 (ebook) | ISBN
   9781718215818 (paperback) | ISBN 9781718215825 (epub) | ISBN
   9781718215832 (pdf)
Subjects: LCSH: Physical fitness for children. | Muscle strength.
Classification: LCC GV443 .V346 2025 (print) | LCC GV443 (ebook) | DDC
   613.7083--dc23/eng/20230801
LC record available at https://lccn.loc.gov/2023031845
LC ebook record available at https://lccn.loc.gov/2023031846

ISBN: 978-1-7182-1581-8 (print)

Copyright © 2025 by Human Kinetics, Inc.

Human Kinetics supports copyright. Copyright fuels scientific and artistic endeavor, encourages authors to create new works, and promotes free speech. Thank you for buying an authorized edition of this work and for complying with copyright laws by not reproducing, scanning, or distributing any part of it in any form without written permission from the publisher. You are supporting authors and allowing Human Kinetics to continue to publish works that increase the knowledge, enhance the performance, and improve the lives of people all over the world.

Notwithstanding the above notice, permission to reproduce the following material is granted to persons and agencies who have purchased this work: pp. 105, 120-140.

The online video and learning content that accompanies this product is delivered on HK*Propel*, **HKPropel. HumanKinetics.com**. You agree that you will not use HK*Propel* if you do not accept the site's Privacy Policy and Terms and Conditions, which detail approved uses of the online content.

To report suspected copyright infringement of content published by Human Kinetics, contact us at **permissions@hkusa.com**. To request permission to legally reuse content published by Human Kinetics, please refer to the information at **https://US.HumanKinetics.com/pages/permissions-information**.

This publication is written and published to provide accurate and authoritative information relevant to the subject matter presented. It is published and sold with the understanding that the author and publisher are not engaged in rendering legal, medical, or other professional services by reason of their authorship or publication of this work. If medical or other expert assistance is required, the services of a competent professional person should be sought.

The web addresses cited in this text were current as of August 2023, unless otherwise noted.

Acquisitions Editor: Mark Manross; **Developmental Editor:** Melissa J. Zavala; **Copyeditor:** Jenny MacKay; **Proofreader:** A.E. Williams; **Permissions Manager:** Laurel Mitchell; **Graphic Designer:** Dawn Sills; **Cover Designer:** Keri Evans; **Cover Design Specialist:** Susan Rothermel Allen; **Photograph (cover):** Hanife Gondogdu; **Photographs (interior):** © Human Kinetics, unless otherwise noted; **Photo Asset Manager:** Laura Fitch; **Photo Production Manager:** Jason Allen; **Senior Art Manager:** Kelly Hendren; **Illustrations:** © Human Kinetics, unless otherwise noted; **Printer:** Versa Press

Printed in the United States of America   10 9 8 7 6 5 4 3 2 1

The paper in this book is certified under a sustainable forestry program.

Human Kinetics
1607 N. Market Street
Champaign, IL 61820
USA

United States and International
Website: **US.HumanKinetics.com**
Email: info@hkusa.com
Phone: 1-800-747-4457

Canada
Website: **Canada.HumanKinetics.com**
Email: info@hkcanada.com

E8792 (paperback)

Contents

Foreword   vii | Preface   ix | Acknowledgments   xiii

PART I Foundations of Functional Strength Training   1

1 Strength Training for All   3
What Is Strength?   5
Strength Training Options   6
What's Next   13

2 Why Functional Strength Training?   15
Benefits of Functional Strength Training   17
What's Next   25

3 Functional Strength Training 101   27
Functional Joint-by-Joint Approach   27
Functional Movement Patterns Versus Muscle Groups   30
Planes of Motion   31
Unilateral Versus Bilateral Exercises   32
Debunking Common Strength Training Myths   34
What's Next   37

4 Functional Strength Training Progressions and Regressions   39
Implementing Skill Progressions and Regressions   40
Example Skill Variations   40
What's Next   43

PART II Functional Strength Training for Physical Education   45

5 Why Functional Strength Training in Physical Education?   47
Benefits of Functional Strength Training in Physical Education   48
Challenges of Implementing Functional Strength Training in Physical Education   48
Tips for Implementing Functional Strength Training   51
What's Next   52

6 Curriculum Design   53
The Victor Way   53
Applying Skill Progressions to a Sequential K-12 Curriculum Map   56
Secondary PE Functional Strength Training Curriculum Outline   57
Using a Curriculum Map to Build a Unit Plan   61
FUNdamentals of Functional Strength Training in Elementary Physical Education   63
Connecting Functional Strength Training to National Standards   68
What's Next   69

7 Teaching Considerations   71
Class Management Strategies   74
Lesson Sequencing   76
Safety Considerations   77
Functional Strength Training and the Affective Domain   78
Modifications for Students With Disabilities   79
What's Next   80

8 Assessment   81
Why Assess?   82
Assessment Types   87
Cognitive Assessment   91
Using Assessments to Calculate Physical Education Grades   92
What's Next   94

PART III Functional Strength Training in Action 95

9 Facility Design 97
Spatial Considerations 97
Equipment Considerations 98
Facility Flow 100
What's Next 102

10 Program Design 103
Exercise Selection 103
Volume 104
Intensity 104
Individualized Modifications Based on Personal Goals and Ability Level 104
What's Next 107

11 Connecting Functional Strength Training in Physical Education to Athletics 109
Goals of a Quality High School Strength and Conditioning Program 109
Extracurricular Sport Performance Program Design Guidelines 110
Strength and Conditioning Certification Recommendations 117
Closing Remarks 118

Appendix: Functional Strength Training for PE Resources 119
Bibliography 141
About the Author 145

Foreword

The Victor Central School Physical Education Department program has been one of the best physical education (PE) programs in New York State as well as in the nation, as recognized by SHAPE America. These recognitions were based on offering unique units, having a comprehensive K-12 curriculum, and having full assessments for every K-12 unit. All Victor PE teachers pride themselves on delivering content based on the K-12 curriculum.

Therefore, it is no surprise that when we were developing our functional strength training unit, it would follow our guidelines of adhering to quality content instruction, and assessments. We were very fortunate to have Nate VanKouwenberg guide our teachers through this process. My role as the director of physical education was to support Nate as he introduced functional strength training to our staff. After meeting with Nate several times, he had me convinced that this was a unit on the cutting edge and that it was going to be extremely beneficial to our students.

How did we get our teachers to buy in to this new unit? We took the time to meet with the entire staff and talk about Nate's goals and objectives for the program. Certainly, some teachers questioned why this unit was necessary, and we had our doubters. The key to the success of the unit was teaching each PE teacher how to perform these skills correctly. When you have teachers who are confident in their abilities to do the specifics of each exercise and teach it to their students, success will follow, and it did!

Nate consistently worked with our teachers to show them the correct technique for all lifts. His passion was contagious! When they had questions, Nate was there each step of the way to help and guide them. After each functional strength training unit, the teachers' confidence grew. As the director of physical education, it was rewarding for me to walk into the fitness room and see our students perform the skills with competency and proficiency. As in the case of all Victor PE units, our students are assessed on their performance, a testament to the skills they have acquired.

Not only did our functional strength training unit teach our students how to perform these exercises safely and proficiently, but the benefits were seen in our athletic teams as well. Our student-athletes are simply stronger and more agile, flexible, and confident than their opponents.

Nate has been a great leader in bringing functional strength training to Victor Central Schools. His passion and commitment to functional strength training and its benefits have made believers of our PE teachers and athletic coaches. Our students and athletes have enthusiastically embraced functional strength training, and so can yours!

Ron Whitcomb
Director of Health, Physical Education, and Athletics (Retired)
Victor Central Schools

Preface

Functional strength training is the latest buzz phrase in fitness, but what is functional strength training, and why is it so important? Recent studies supporting the importance of functional strength for all populations cannot be ignored. To achieve personal goals connected to daily activities and general health, strength training with a purpose should be at the forefront of every fitness program. Whether the goal is to improve body composition, physical performance, or long-term durability, functional strength training can provide the best bang for the buck when compared with traditional isolation-based strength training and constant-state cardio.

If functional strength training can drastically improve quality of life, longevity, and performance, why are more people not incorporating these methods into their weekly fitness regimens? In most cases, they may not know where to start, they may have misconceptions about strength training in general, or it may be a combination of both.

What better way to introduce functional strength training to the masses than in physical education (PE)? The fact that most U.S. states and many countries mandate some form of physical education for all students provides PE teachers with the unique opportunity to introduce functional strength training on a global scale.

Despite the amazing opportunity PE teachers have to introduce quality functional strength training to youths, far too many fitness units in PE classes are stuck decades behind the times by placing an emphasis on machine-based isolation strength training, or even worse, no strength training at all. By learning how to perform functional skills with proper technique and to design quality workouts connected to their personal goals, students will have the tools required to build a strong foundation of wellness for a lifetime.

Students deserve to be exposed to the most up-to-date fitness activities, even if it requires teachers to go outside of their comfort zones to bring themselves up to speed. This is the time to spark a change in the quality of fitness units in PE classes by providing teachers with the basic knowledge and skills required to introduce functional strength training to children and adolescents all over the world!

Why I Wrote This Book

As a young PE teacher, I knew that I wanted to pursue strength and conditioning outside of school in some capacity after catching the bug for quality functional fitness in college. What started as a side hustle training a few high school hockey players at a local gym during school breaks grew to a well-respected functional fitness and sport performance company called Next Level Strength and Conditioning in Rochester, New York. Now, almost 20 years later, I have had the privilege of working with countless high school, college, and professional athletes along with some of the best strength coaches in the industry. In addition to my role as the owner of Next Level, I have served as the strength coach for the Rochester Institute of Technology Division 1 men's hockey team and the strength and conditioning coordinator at Victor Central Schools in New York, where I also teach physical education at the junior high school to this day. My intention behind listing my professional accomplishments is not to pump my own tires but to emphasize how my inability to sit still has provided me with a long résumé in the functional fitness, sport performance, and PE fields.

Early in my teaching career, I took the lead on revamping my school district's fitness curriculum to apply my strength and conditioning experience to what we were doing in physical education. With the help of my amazing colleagues at Victor, we were able to swap outdated fitness methods for the latest in functional strength training. It didn't take long to realize that we were on to something special that was making a huge impact on our students.

When other districts caught wind of what we were doing in our PE fitness units, I began to receive requests to present at New York State Association for Health, Physical Education, Recreation and Dance conferences and neighboring districts' professional development workshops. It was obvious to me right off the bat that a shocking number of PE teachers were in dire need of direction to update their current offerings with functional strength training. After several years of presenting on this topic, I have helped many fellow educators make drastic changes to their programs. Now, I am honored to compile my experiences in this step-by-step manual that will provide teachers with a one-stop-shop resource to take their PE fitness units to the next level.

Functional Strength Training for PE Overview

This book was developed to provide a detailed and easy-to-follow manual for PE teachers who would like to implement functional strength training into their fitness units. Regardless of grade level, unique circumstances, or previous experience in this area, teachers will be able to navigate through the four main parts of this comprehensive guide with ease.

Part I: Foundations of Functional Strength Training

The first part of this book focuses on the content knowledge associated with functional strength training, which will allow teachers to understand the *why* behind the concepts they will be teaching in class. In what I refer to as "Functional Strength Training 101," teachers will receive a summary of important topics including the benefits of functional strength training, general terminology, common misconceptions, skill progressions, and more.

Part II: Functional Strength Training for Physical Education

In this section, I use nearly 20 years of experience in both the fitness and PE fields to tailor these overarching concepts to the classroom setting. This section will provide you with a comprehensive guide to curriculum design, teaching considerations, modifications for special populations, and assessment, specific to functional strength training in physical education at all levels.

Part III: Functional Strength Training in Action

The third part of this book takes a deep dive into functional strength training beyond the classroom, because ultimately, what we want for students is to continue participating in functional strength training independently in order to achieve lifetime wellness and reach their personal goals. In this section, I review a wide range of topics that will help PE teachers provide students with opportunities to apply what they learn in class on their own time, including facility design considerations, functional strength training program design guidelines, and advanced functional strength training for performance and athletics.

Functional Strength Training for PE Resources

The appendix includes resources required for PE teachers to successfully design and implement quality functional strength training units and extracurricular activities, regardless of previous experience and knowledge in this area. This section includes external skill cues, a sample curriculum map, a personalized curriculum design template, assessment checklists, sample functional strength training, and sport performance programs. Downloadable versions of the appendix material are available in HK*Propel*. These forms may be used as-is or modified to fit the needs of individual programs. HK*Propel* also offers photographs and videos of exercise demonstrations. Teachers will be able to use these photos and video demonstrations to gain confidence in their own ability to teach functional skills in class and may project these photos or videos during class to demonstrate skills.

See the card at the front of the print book for your unique HK*Propel* access code. For ebook users, reference the HK*Propel* access code instructions on the page immediately following the book cover.

Acknowledgments

To Ash, Rea, and B.: Thank you for your unwavering love and support. Out of all the hats I wear, I am most proud of "Father" and "Husband." It's all for you.

To T.V.K. and Frances: Thank you for building the foundation of our family on God, love, and hard work. Sara, Em, and I would not be where we are today without you as our role models.

To my Victor PE colleagues, past and present: Thank you for taking so much pride in our profession and for going above and beyond to do what's best for kids. I am proud to be a member of this PE all-star team.

To our team of stud Next Level coaches, especially Mooner, Bricks, Joey, and Haley: Thank you for caring as much as you do and for running the show while I took a step back to complete this project. We wouldn't be here without you.

To Erika Insalaco: Thank you for taking the time to review my work and for not charging me per comma.

PART I

Foundations of Functional Strength Training

Chapters 1 through 4 focus on the content knowledge associated with functional strength training, which will allow teachers to understand the "why" behind the concepts they will be teaching in class. In what is referred to as "Functional Strength Training 101," teachers will receive a summary of important topics including the benefits of functional strength training, general terminology, common misconceptions, skill progressions, and more.

1

Strength Training for All

Most people start workout programs, join gyms, or hire personal trainers to improve how they look, feel, perform, and to live long, healthy lives. The good news is that there has been a significant increase in fitness and healthy nutrition options for the general public in recent years. The bad news is that the average person without a background in fitness and nutrition is being bombarded with misinformation, resulting in wasted time, delayed benefits, and even the risk of injury.

When most people decide it's time to get in shape, they may start running or join a gym packed wall to wall with cardio equipment and isolation-based selectorized machines. Hats off to anyone who makes the decision to take steps toward self-improvement, but there are important factors to consider before deciding on an approach.

> "You don't run to get fit; you need to be fit to run."
> —Diane Lee

- Is long-distance running a safe option for average people early in their fitness journeys? Many qualified fitness professionals would argue that it is not. Although there are tremendous cardiovascular and energy-balance benefits that come with distance running, it can take a toll on joints, especially the knees, if a base foundation of strength is lacking (U.S. National Library of Medicine 2020). It is no surprise that many people are forced to stop running before their fitness goals are reached due to knee issues when strength is ignored.

- There is nothing wrong with cardio machines such as treadmills, ellipticals, arc trainers, and stationary bikes. These are all much better options than riding the couch, and cardiovascular health and energy balance are critical ingredients in the recipe for lifelong wellness. However, there is so much more that needs to be addressed. Spending most of your time on cardio equipment without strength training is like making a pizza without the crust. A solid foundation needs to be in place to support the rest of life's activities.

- One of the biggest barriers to participating in a regular fitness program is time. People are busy, and exercise often takes a back seat to the rest of life's obligations. Unfortunately, just walking into the gym and checking the box doesn't get you any closer to your goals. If you only have a small slice of time in your day to knock out a quick workout, don't you want to get the best bang for your buck? If forced to choose between 30 minutes on a piece of cardio equipment or 30 minutes with a few free weights, I would pick the free weights 100% of the time, not only because of the versatility of free weights but because the average jaunt on a cardio machine does not compare to the comprehensive benefit of a quality full-body strength workout (Gustavo et al. 2018).

According to an article published on the Harvard Health Blog in May 2015 that outlined the findings of an international study conducted from 2003 to 2009, "Grip strength is a better predictor of death or cardiovascular disease than blood pressure" (LeWine 2015, 4). Similar research findings, published in *The Lancet* (Leong et al. 2015), came from the international Prospective Urban Rural Epidemiology (PURE) study.

Here's a breakdown of that study and its findings:

- Grip strength was measured using a dynamometer in nearly 140,000 adults in 17 countries while monitoring the health of participants over the course of 4 years.
- Each 11 lb (5 kg) decrease in grip strength over the course of the study was linked to a 16% higher risk of dying from any cause, a 17% higher risk of dying from heart disease, a 9% higher risk of a stroke, and a 7% higher risk of a heart attack.
- Connections between grip strength, death, and cardiovascular disease remained strong even after researchers adjusted for other factors such as age, smoking, and exercise.
- The study concluded that grip strength was a better predictor of death or cardiovascular disease than was blood pressure.

Why did the researchers choose grip strength as the measuring stick for this study? Most likely, it was because of the reliability, validity, and availability of dynamometers. Additionally, a strong correlation exists between grip strength and nervous system function, which plays a major role in overall wellness and longevity. Although the study did state that "further research is needed to identify determinants of muscular strength and to test whether improvements in strength reduce mortality and cardiovascular disease" (Leong et al. 2015, 266), this is still a big win for those of us in the "strength matters" camp.

The following excerpts from the article on the Harvard Health Blog (LeWine 2015) also link grip strength to biological age:

An individual's age in years (chronological age) can be quite different from his or her biological age. Although there's no exact definition for biological age, it generally indicates whether the body is functioning better or worse than its chronological age (7).

The researchers suggest that weaker muscle strength makes it more likely that a person will die sooner if he or she develops a chronic medical problem, compared with those who have more muscle strength. In other words, muscle strength could be good for survival (10).

Mic drop! Strength clearly needs to be a priority for all.

What Is Strength?

As defined in *The Merriam-Webster Dictionary*, strength is the "capacity for exertion or endurance" or "the ability to resist being moved or broken by a force." Note that there is nothing in the definition about bench day or getting "swole." If we dive deeper into this definition, it sounds a lot like what most people are hoping to get out of their fitness program.

- *Capacity for exertion or endurance.* Strength provides a solid foundation that will support demanding physical activities and sports for extended periods of time.
- *Ability to resist being moved or broken by a force.* Strength increases durability, which can protect people against the inevitable dangers of life and prepare them for daily physical tasks and sports for all ages.
  - "Strong people are harder to kill and more useful in general."—Mark Rippetoe
- *A strong foundation.* For people interested in improving physical performance, a solid foundation of strength will maximize the development and expression of speed, agility, and power (Seitz et al. 2014). I would much rather build my house on a solid concrete foundation than a sand beach.
  - "You can't fire a cannon from a canoe!"—Charles Poliquin

Unfortunately, countless people are missing out on the benefits of strength training because they

- don't understand the true benefits or don't think they need strength to reach their goals;
- don't know where to start due to lack of previous exposure, knowledge, and skill; or
- lack confidence due to a distorted view of strength training, thanks to countless fitness myths and the old-school "meathead" culture.

Let's address each of these potential hurdles.

- The benefits of strength training apply to people of all ages, regardless of individualized goals and needs (Westcott 2012), and include the following:
    - Longevity and durability
    - Bone density
    - Boosted metabolism and improvements in healthy body composition (increased muscle mass results in a small increase in the basal metabolic rate, or energy used at rest)
    - Physical performance
    - Aesthetics of lean muscle mass
    - Confidence and self-esteem
    - Improved cognitive function and mood
- Performing a handful of basic resistance exercises 2 to 4 days each week will go a long way. Strength training does not need to be fancy, complicated, or at world-record intensities to be effective. Strength is relative. While a 400 lb (181 kg) deadlift may be an appropriate intensity for an elite athlete, a 40 lb (18 kg) deadlift may be equally challenging for a 70-year-old grandparent.
- The thought of strength training may be intimidating for people who have visions of muscle-bound hunks grunting and throwing weights around the gym. It's time to shift the narrative surrounding strength training to debunk decades of misconceptions.

The good news for the cardio lovers out there is that you don't need to pick between strength training and cardiovascular activities. A comprehensive fitness program should include 2 to 4 days of strength training each week, in addition to cardiovascular exercise and a wide variety of other physical activities that people enjoy.

Strength Training Options

Now that I'm blue in the face after preaching about the importance of strength training for the masses, where do we go from here? Although strength training does not need to be complicated to make a major impact, there are several things that need to be considered before jumping into a strength training program. What exercises should you pick? How many repetitions should you do and how much weight should you use? What about that (fill in the blank) injury from a few years ago? These are all valid questions that often freeze strength training newbies in their tracks due to paralysis by analysis. It's much easier to just jump on the elliptical machine.

All of these topics will be addressed in later chapters, but let's start with the strength training options available and a general overview of each. Table 1.1 summarizes each option, including a brief description, benefits, possible negatives, and the equipment required.

Table 1.1 **Summary of Strength Training Options**

Strength training option	Description	Benefits	Possible negatives	Equipment
Functional strength training	Multijoint exercises; realistic movement patterns	Benefits daily activities and general fitness goals	Requires a base level of knowledge, skill, and ability	Body weight, free weights, etc.
Isolation strength training	Targets one muscle group at a time	Requires little knowledge, skill, and ability; hypertrophy	Not as applicable to daily activities; increased time	Machines, free weights, bands
Powerlifting	Competitive sport; includes back squat, bench press, and deadlift	Incorporates functional exercises	Maximum intensity is not always connected to goals; increased risk of injury	Barbells, weighted plates, squat racks, benches
Olympic weightlifting	Competitive sport: snatch, clean and jerk	Increased power, speed, coordination, and force absorption	Exercises are very technical; increased risk of injury	Barbells, Olympic bumper plates
CrossFit	High-intensity functional training	Community; increased functional fitness	Increased risk of injury if not scaled for individualized needs	Body weight, free weights, barbells, variety of plates, etc.

Functional Strength Training

Functional strength training is strength training with a purpose. Exercises use multiple muscle groups simultaneously in realistic movement patterns that will benefit daily activities and increase longevity (figure 1.1).

Benefits

- The benefits of functional strength training far outweigh those of other types of strength training for the average person and athlete (Stenger 2018) due to the direct correlation between functional movement patterns and daily activities. Several other advantages unique to functional strength training will be discussed in detail throughout this book.

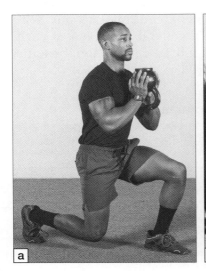 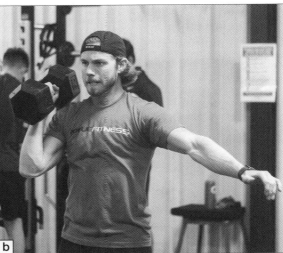

Figure 1.1 Functional exercises: *(a)* goblet split squat and *(b)* dumbbell 1-arm overhead press.
(b) Hanife Gondogdu

Possible Negatives
- Functional strength training requires a base level of knowledge, skill, and ability, which may become a barrier for people just getting started. This is why functional strength training needs to be introduced to children in PE classes all over the world.

Equipment and Space Required
- Minimal equipment and space are needed for functional strength training. Functional exercises can be performed with body weight or with a variety of free weights and other implements that will be discussed in later chapters.

Isolation Strength Training

Isolation strength training targets one muscle group at a time. This is a traditional form of strength training that has been a staple in large corporate gyms and PE fitness units for decades (figure 1.2).

Benefits
- This form of strength training may be more appealing for people with less experience because it requires very little skill, knowledge, and ability.
- Isolation strength training can increase hypertrophy, which is ideal for bodybuilders and athletes who would like to add muscle mass for additional body armor.
- Strength training using selectorized machines may provide a safe alternative to people with physical limitations.

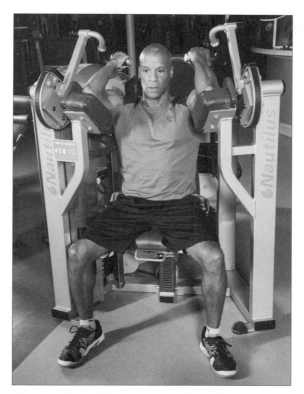

Figure 1.2 Isolation selectorized machines have been a staple in strength training for decades.

Possible Negatives

- Isolation training develops segmental strength, which is not as realistic to how the body moves in daily activities and sports when compared to functional strength.
- Less gets done in more time. Targeting one muscle group at a time with little to no core engagement or cardiovascular demand significantly increases the amount of time required to complete a comprehensive, full-body workout.
- Selectorized machines are expensive, take up a lot of space, and guide the user through the movement, limiting neuromuscular demand, joint-stability benefits, and core engagement.

Equipment and Space Required

- Isolation training requires free weights, bands, and selectorized machines.

Powerlifting

Powerlifting is a competitive sport in which participants attempt to lift maximal loads in the back squat, bench press, and deadlift. Although these exercises are all functional in nature, the primary objective of powerlifting is to lift as much weight as possible (figure 1.3).

Benefits

- The squat, bench press, and deadlift are foundational compound movements that should be a major component of most general-population strength training and athletic development programs to improve function, performance, and durability.

Possible Negatives

- The lines between lifting as much weight as possible and the benefits of performing these exercises correctly while gradually increasing weight are often blurred. This can lead to athletes sacrificing performance in their sport to chase numbers in the weight room. General fitness participants who obsess about the amount of weight on the bar instead of their true goals are also putting themselves at major risk of injury. The goal of the squat, bench press, and deadlift for athletes and

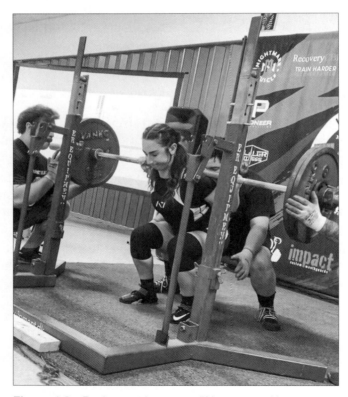

Figure 1.3 Back squat in a powerlifting competition.

the average person should be to perform each movement with proper form through the full range of motion while gradually increasing resistance, not to set world records. As the legendary strength coach Dan John says, "The goal is to keep the goal the goal."

Equipment and Space Required
- Powerlifting requires barbells, weighted plates, benches, and squat racks.

Olympic Weightlifting

Olympic weightlifting, in which men and women attempt to lift as much weight as possible over their heads in two exercises called the *snatch* and the *clean and jerk*, has been an Olympic sport since 1920. These full-body, multijoint exercises are explosive, requiring participants to move submaximal loads at high rates of velocity (figure 1.4).

Benefits
- Variations of the snatch and the clean and jerk (including the hang snatch, dumbbell snatch, hang clean, hang power clean, and many others) are often embedded within advanced sport-performance

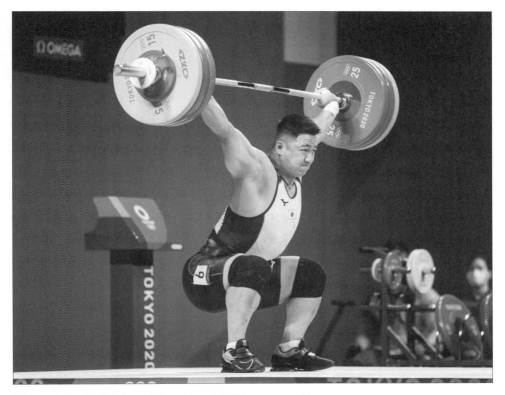

Figure 1.4 Snatch in an Olympic weightlifting competition.
Tom Weller/DeFodi Images via Getty Images Images / Contributor

training programs because when they are performed correctly, they increase power, speed, coordination, and the ability to absorb force.

Possible Negatives
- Olympic weightlifting is the most technical form of strength training. A great deal of physical ability and skill development with meaningful progressions is required to perform the exercises safely. Even the most seasoned Olympic weightlifting veterans put themselves at risk of injury when performing these exercises. Athletes and the average person with general fitness goals must weigh the risk-to-benefit ratio when considering Olympic weightlifting and related variations.

Equipment and Space Required
- Olympic weightlifting uses barbells and Olympic bumper plates.

CrossFit

CrossFit is a branded fitness regimen founded in 2000 by Greg and Lauren Glassman, and it combines a wide variety of functional training methods. This mix of general functional strength training, powerlifting, Olympic weightlifting, gymnastics, and high-intensity interval training (HIIT) is often referred to as high-intensity functional training (HIFT). The community aspect of CrossFit took the world by storm in the early 2000s, introducing functional training to people of all ages and backgrounds (figure 1.5). The CrossFit Games incorporate intense functional training methods into fitness competitions, ultimately naming the "Fittest Man and Woman on Earth."

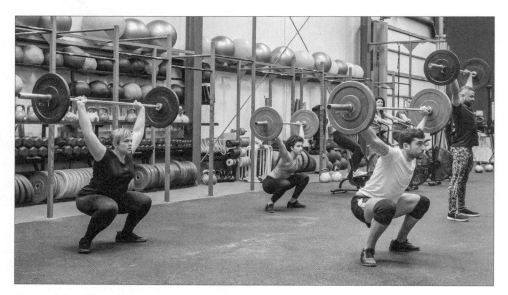

Figure 1.5 Olympic snatch in a CrossFit class.
doble-d/iStock/Getty Images

Benefits
- The community aspect and branding of CrossFit have helped make functional training mainstream over the past 20 years. When CrossFit workouts are programmed with sound progressions, individualized modifications, and safe volume and intensity, participants may experience the health and performance results of a comprehensive functional training program.

Possible Negatives
- Although CrossFit has made a major effort to prioritize safety and individualization in recent years, many fitness professionals have scrutinized its training methods in the past, due to reports of training-related injuries in the media. Even though this is not unique to CrossFit, the safety of each participant must be the number one priority when strength training. Individualized needs, ability level, experience, volume, and intensity must be considered when performing technical functional exercises. It is critical that CrossFit coaches stress the difference between CrossFit (the scalable fitness regimen) and the CrossFit Games (the sport of fitness) to prevent average fitness enthusiasts from trying to keep up with the fittest people on the planet. However, despite the possible safety concerns, recent studies have been unable to prove that CrossFit training is more dangerous than traditional strength training modalities (Feito, Burrows, and Tabb 2018).

Equipment and Space Required
- CrossFit gyms, or "boxes," traditionally include a minimal open-space format with a wide range of functional training equipment.

What's Next

Now that we have established the importance of strength training for all and have clearly defined the different options to consider, let's take a closer look at functional strength training. Not only will we discuss the long list of benefits that come with functional strength training, but real-life examples will be provided to further plead the case that this form of fitness should be a priority for people of all ages.

2

Why Functional Strength Training?

Let's take a deeper dive into functional strength training, or simply put, training with a purpose. The *Oxford English Dictionary* defines the word *functional* as

- having a special activity, purpose, or task; relating to the way in which something works or operates, or
- designed to be practical and useful, rather than attractive.

When applied to strength training and exercise, these definitions highlight how functional strength training is intended to benefit daily activities and tasks based on how the body operates. My wife went to college for interior design, and she is constantly moving things in our house around, telling me how the current arrangement of furniture makes our living space more functional. Is the functional place for a grill in your backyard or your bathroom? Although a grill in the bathroom might sound like a dream come true for some, you get the point. If strength training using multiple muscle groups simultaneously in realistic patterns is like having your grill in the backyard, then sitting down on a machine using one muscle at a time is like grilling in the bathroom. It doesn't make much sense.

When *functional strength training* became a new buzz term in the early 2000s, some people overassociated balance and instability with this new trend. Like many other people at the time, I thought that if I added a stability ball or BOSU ball to any exercise, it would make it more "functional." I'm embarrassed to admit that as a young strength coach in the early 2000s, I would even have athletes do curls on a BOSU ball! Mike Boyle, one of the pioneers of functional strength training, released his first edition of *Functional Training for Sports* in 2003. Anyone who knows or follows Coach Boyle today would be floored to know that the cover of his first book (figure 2.1a) pictures an athlete on a balance board! Things have

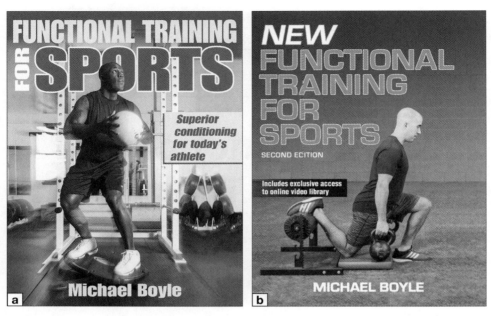

Figure 2.1 Book covers for Mike Boyle's *(a) Functional Training for Sports* and *(b) New Functional Training for Sports*.

clearly come a long way over the past 20 years. Coach Boyle released *New Functional Training for Sports* in 2016 with an athlete performing a rear foot elevated split squat on the cover (figure 2.1b). Now that's more like it!

What Makes Training Functional?

- Using multiple muscle groups simultaneously in realistic movement patterns
    - Squat
    - Lunge
    - Hip hinge
    - Upper body push (horizontal or vertical)
    - Upper body pull (horizontal or vertical)
    - Rotation
    - Core stability
- Performing exercises in all planes of motion
    - Sagittal
    - Frontal
    - Transverse

- Incorporating exercises that require realistic coordination, stability, and eccentric demands
  - Unilateral or single-leg exercises
  - Using free weights and other implements that require motor control, core engagement, balance, and joint stability
  - Jumping, leaping, and hopping with an extra emphasis on proper landing mechanics

Benefits of Functional Strength Training

When people ask for my thoughts on one of the countless fitness options available, my boilerplate response is always in question format: Is it safe and pain-free? Do you enjoy it enough to get out of bed in the morning or exercise after work? Is it helping you reach your goals? If the answer is *yes* to all three questions, I think that method of exercise is a solid choice. However, as I mentioned before, there are several benefits that are exclusive to functional strength training. Here is a detailed list of reasons why I would strongly recommend incorporating functional strength training in some capacity 2 to 4 days a week, regardless of age, ability level, or personal goals.

Support for Daily Activities and Physical Tasks

I'll say it one more time—functional strength training benefits daily activities and tasks because exercises are performed in realistic movement patterns. As an example, how many times have you heard someone say, "Lift with your legs, not your back?" We all know that picking up heavy objects by bending at the waist with a rounded back is dangerous and can lead to long-term injury. Lifting a heavy object off the ground correctly with a flat back looks a lot like the deadlift or hip hinge movement pattern (figure 2.2). Learning how to correctly hinge at the hip while building a solid foundation of strength in this pattern will correlate to daily life much better than separating all of the muscle groups involved and training them individually. Does it make more sense to perform 3 to 5 sets of an appropriate deadlift variation or to sit on the hamstring curl, leg extension, abdominal crunch, and back extension machines separately to target only some of the muscle groups involved in this common daily task? When viewed this way, common sense usually prevails. This is only one of endless examples of how functional strength training in realistic movement patterns is more beneficial and efficient than isolation-based strength training.

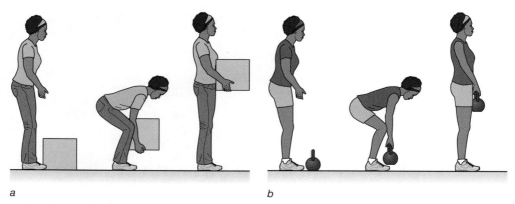

Figure 2.2 Comparison between *(a)* daily tasks and *(b)* the deadlift.

Reduced Injury

It is impossible to guarantee that any precautionary measure will prevent injury. Freak accidents happen in life and in sports, no matter what you do in the gym. With that said, quality functional strength training has been proven to reduce the risk of injury (Lauersen, Bertelsen, and Andersen 2013). As mentioned previously, general strength will improve overall durability regardless of preferred training methods, but the additional perks of functional strength training will further decrease the risk of injury in life and sports. Performing multijoint movements with free weights and other implements that require coordination, balance, and eccentric control in multiple planes of motion will drastically improve joint stability and functional symmetry (Behm and Colado 2012). People who strength train on machines are missing out on valuable proprioception (the body's ability to sense its location and movement in space) and neuromuscular system benefits, because machines guide the user through the movement in a singular plane of motion. In everyday life and sports, reactive stability and deceleration in multiple planes of motion are required. Improving functional symmetry will also improve how joints and corresponding muscle groups work together to decrease the likelihood of breakdown and overuse injuries caused by common functional imbalances.

Enhanced Sport Performance

Just like daily physical tasks, sports and other performance-based physical activities are performed with multiple joints working together in all planes of motion. Most sports are played on one leg at a time and require athletes to produce and absorb force rapidly in environments full of variable external factors that can change in a split second. Does this sound like sitting on a machine and using one muscle group at a time? Functional strength training is one of the primary building blocks used when designing a program to improve sport performance. To increase strength, power, speed, agility, and endurance that can be applied to sports, athletes must consistently incorporate compound movements with authentic neuromuscular system demands in their comprehensive training programs (Xiao et al. 2021). In sport performance training, we have seen a major shift over the past 2 decades from isolation-based selectorized machines and long-distance, constant-state cardio to functional strength training, sprinting, jumping, and interval-based training. This shift has resulted in elite athletes changing the face of sports due to their unprecedented physical ability (figure 2.3).

As an incoming freshman college hockey player in the late 1990s, I had no idea how to prepare for my first season of collegiate athletics, so I did what my friends were doing. For the next 4 months, I went to the gym religiously. I would split up my training days by separating muscle groups, usually on machines, and would always finish with 100 crunches and a 3 mi (5 km) run. I put on more than 10 lb (5 kg) of muscle and thought I was in the best shape of my life. I was wrong. I will never forget how slow and out of shape I felt on the ice when I got to school and started skating with the team. After almost getting cut as a recruited freshman, I realized

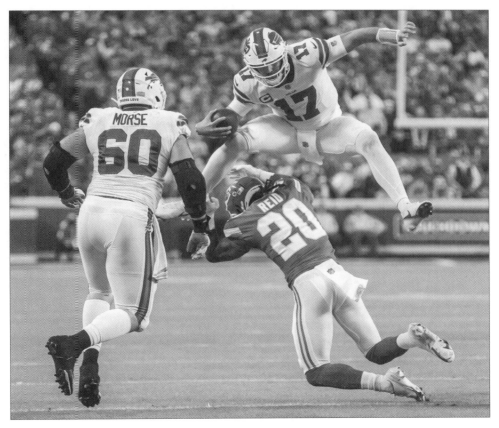

Figure 2.3 Josh Allen hurdling over a Kansas City Chiefs player.
Nick Tre. Smith/Icon Sportswire via Getty Images
Icon Sportswire / Contributor

I needed to do something different for the next off-season. This is when I was introduced to Mike Boyle and functional strength training. A former teammate of mine, Dave Insalaco, trained at Mike Boyle Strength and Conditioning after his first year of playing professionally. The following off-season when he returned home for the summer, we became training partners. I went from doing seated biceps curls, triceps extensions, and long-distance runs to split squats, lateral lunges, single-leg deadlifts, plyometrics, short sprints, a wide variety of functional upper body exercises, and so much more. I didn't spend more time in the gym that off-season, but the results were incomparable. I felt like a completely different athlete and player when it was time to step back on the ice. I remember giggling at myself after making a quick lateral move or blowing someone's doors off in a puck race, because I was so shocked at how different I felt. To say I was inspired and hooked is a blatant understatement. From that point on, I knew that my career was going to be something in the field of fitness and sport performance.

Now, over 20 years later, sport performance training resources are widespread. However, when it comes to applying functional strength training to sports, I can't recommend Mike Boyle's book *New Functional Training for Sports* (2016) highly enough. Although we will discuss the application of functional strength training for sport performance in the school setting throughout this book, I suggest referring to *New Functional Training for Sports* to learn more about the application of functional strength training to sport performance.

Correct Posture

As if posture hasn't always been important for function, performance, and injury reduction, now we have to deal with "text neck," or upper cross syndrome (UCS). Our societal addiction to technology and handheld devices, paired with an increase in desk jobs and sedentary lifestyles, has literally changed the physical composition of our population at an alarming rate (Karimian et al. 2019). A constant forward head posture while looking at handheld devices and sitting at a desk all day cause weak neck flexors, tight chest muscles, weak midback muscles, and tight upper back muscles. This combination can drastically affect the resting posture of the head, neck, and back. In extreme cases, UCS can lead to changes in the position of the cervical spine, causing the head to sit forward in front of the neck at rest. There are reports that the head feels like it weighs about 10 lb (5kg) when it sits on top of the neck with proper posture and almost 60 lb (27 kg) in extreme cases of UCS (David et al. 2021) (figure 2.4). That's bananas! So, what can we do? Aside from using handheld devices in moderation, increasing time on our feet, and making conscious changes to our resting posture, consistent functional strength training can help both correct and prevent "text neck." A comprehensive functional training program should include a balanced ratio of upper body pulling and upper

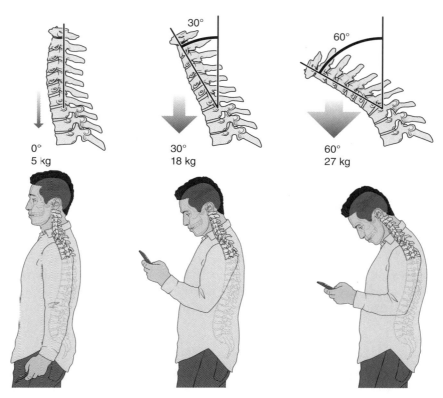

Figure 2.4 When flexed forward on the neck, the weight of the head is drastically increased.

body pushing exercises. Improving midback strength with a wide variety of upper body pulling exercises, without overemphasizing upper body pushing movements, will help "open up" the resting posture. Traditional isolation-based workout programs tend to overdo it on the "beach muscles," which are mainly on the anterior chain, including the pectorals, deltoids, biceps, and abdominals. Over-development of these muscle groups without paying adequate attention to the posterior chain will amplify a hunched-over resting posture. A balanced upper body pull-to-push exercise ratio (or even a 2:1 pull-to-push ratio) along with a steady dose of loaded carries to improve postural integrity under load will do wonders in the fight against "text neck" and poor resting posture.

Improved Body Composition

The term *body composition* refers to the ratio of healthy body mass (muscles, bones, connective tissue, organs, etc.) to fat. There are several tests that can provide body composition scores, including skin fold measurements, hydrostatic weighing, DEXA (bone density) scanning, body mass index (BMI), and more. Some tests are more valid and reliable than others, but they all aim to provide a measurement that compares healthy body mass to fat. Although fat is necessary for the body to function properly, it is no secret that excessive amounts can lead to a wide range of serious health issues.

A large factor in maintaining a healthy body composition is energy balance (calories in versus calories out) (Hill, Wyatt, and Peters 2012). If people consistently ingest more calories (energy) than they burn (energy used to fuel physical activity and general bodily functions) for extended periods, unused calories will be stored as fat. This is known as a calorie surplus. On the flip side, if people consistently ingest fewer calories than they burn, stored fat and even muscle may be used for fuel. This is known as a calorie deficit. Although there are other factors that may play a role, including age, gender, hormones, and genetics, the key to achieving a healthy body composition is maintaining a balanced ratio of calories in versus calories out on a regular basis (figure 2.5).

What does this have to do with functional strength training? As mentioned previously, an increase in muscle mass will result in a small increase in the basal metabolic rate, or energy used at rest. In addition, using multiple large muscle groups simultaneously while performing compound

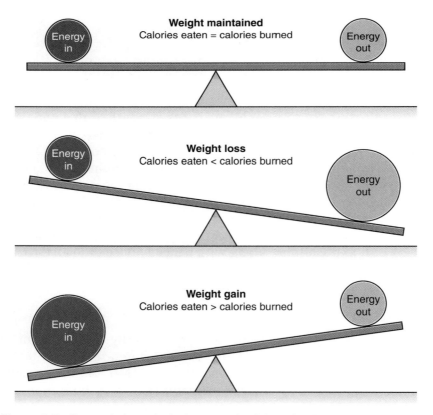

Figure 2.5 Energy balance is the key to maintaining a healthy body composition.

functional exercises will increase the heart rate due to the extra demand for oxygenated blood. This is like a buy one, get one free deal at the local supermarket. Functional strength training will increase healthy muscle mass while burning extra calories due to training at an elevated heart rate. You can't afford not to buy it! When paired with regular cardiovascular exercise and proper nutrition, functional strength training can play a major role in achieving a healthy body composition.

Increased Mobility

Joint mobility refers to the ability to move certain joints through a full range of motion to maximize function and performance. We will take a deeper dive into mobility, the joint-by-joint approach, and common myths surrounding flexibility in later chapters, but one major advantage to consistent functional strength training is improved flexibility and joint mobility (Leite et al. 2017). Isolation-based strength training may decrease mobility because it promotes segmental strength and hypertrophy. However, functional strength training consists of exercises that are performed through a full range of motion, which will have a positive impact on joint mobility over time. Here are just a few examples:

- Squatting through the full range of motion may improve ankle and hip mobility (figure 2.6).
- Vertical, or overhead, pressing with proper form may improve shoulder mobility (figure 2.7).

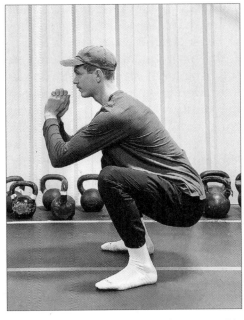

Figure 2.6 Deep squats can improve ankle and hip mobility (original picture).

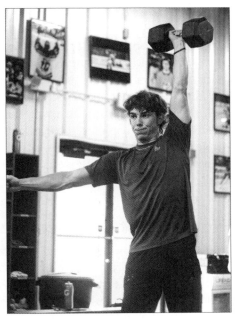

Figure 2.7 Overhead pressing can improve shoulder mobility.
Hanife Gondogdu

- Horizontal pulling, or rowing, exercises may improve thoracic mobility by promoting an open posture and midback strength (figure 2.8).

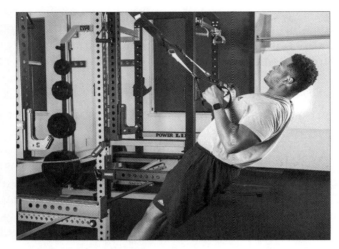

Figure 2.8 Horizontal pulling exercises such as the TRX row can improve thoracic mobility.

Time Saved

Why do so many people flood department stores at the wee hours of the morning on Black Friday to complete the bulk of their holiday shopping? There may be a select few who enjoy the commotion of wrestling over the last flat-screen TV, but I assume most are trying to maximize their purchases. People are able to stretch their hard-earned money, so they jump at the opportunity to get more for less. If time were a form of currency (it could be argued that time is the most valuable asset someone could possess), people should think of functional strength training as the Black Friday of fitness. If there's an option to get more accomplished in less time, why not jump at the opportunity? The benefits of gaining strength in multiple muscle groups while simultaneously using realistic movement patterns through a full range of motion, with the added perks of core engagement, neuromuscular demand, and training at an elevated heart rate, make sitting on a machine that isolates muscle groups seem like a silly waste of valuable time.

Promotion of Confidence and Self-Esteem

The mental, emotional, and social benefits of fitness are often undervalued. Not only are there chemical and hormonal responses to exercise that have positive impacts on mood and behavior (Sharma, Madaan, and Petty 2006), but consistent participation in a strength training program will often improve confidence, self-esteem, and body image as well. I've lost count over the years of how many people I have seen make complete personal transformations after just a few months of consistently buying into a functional strength training program. After realizing what they're capable of in the weight room, people can flip their self-image. This can be life changing! Learning a new movement, performing a chin-up for the first time, or achieving a personal best on a big lift often radiates confidence into other areas of life. Functional strength training offers a unique opportunity for people to achieve self-actualization with the added benefit of improving how they look, feel, and perform.

What's Next

Now that we have established the importance of consistent functional strength training for all ages and ability levels, chapter 3 will take a closer look into the small details that make this form of exercise so beneficial.

3

Functional Strength Training 101

Now that we have established the importance of consistent functional strength training for all ages and ability levels, let's take a deeper dive into the nuts and bolts that make this form of exercise so beneficial.

Functional Joint-by-Joint Approach

As mentioned in the previous chapters, functional strength training consists of multijoint resistance exercises performed in realistic movement patterns. To maximize the benefits of this form of strength training, it's important to know the true function or purpose of each joint. As if the body wasn't amazing enough already, the way joints work in symphony to maximize performance and durability is fascinating. Joints are stacked on top of each other, starting at the ground with the big toe and going all the way up a chain to the upper neck. The function of each joint alternates between mobility and stability as you travel up the chain (Boyle 2016). This concept and how it relates to functional strength training is known as the joint-by-joint approach (figure 3.1).

According to Mike Boyle in his book *New Functional Training for Sports* (2016), the joint-by-joint idea started with an informal conversation between Boyle and a legendary physical therapist, Gray Cook. While discussing results they had seen in Cook's functional movement screen, Cook pointed out that the body is a stack of joints, each with a specific function, which makes levels of dysfunction predictable. The joint-by-joint approach uses common dysfunction issues to target the specific needs of each joint in functional training programs, which can reduce the risk of injury and long-term breakdown.

Except for direct trauma to an area, pain in a joint is usually the symptom of dysfunction in a joint above or below the site of discomfort. For example, when someone has knee pain, it is often caused by compensatory

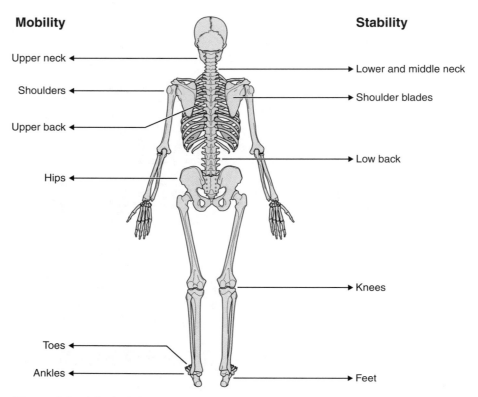

Figure 3.1 Joint-by-joint concept.

patterns that result from a lack of mobility in the ankle or hip. If you had a rope tied to your neck and someone yanked the rope, it would obviously hurt your neck, but the pain in your neck would be caused by the person pulling the rope, not an issue with your neck. Therefore, instead of applying ice for temporary pain relief, the long-term solution would be to get the person to stop pulling on the rope.

When my girls were younger, they had a pink potty step in our bathroom (figure 3.2). One day, I noticed some of the screws on the step were coming loose, but fixing it was far from the top of my list. It slipped my mind until a few weeks later when I came into the bathroom to find that not only were the screws completely removed, but now the hinge on the opposite side was hanging on for dear life. As I stood over this pile of pink particleboard, contemplating whether to put it out of its misery or get a screwdriver, I noticed how well this once fully functional stairway to the porcelain throne related to movement and the human body. The hinge on the bottom right side of the step was minding its own business until the screws on the upper left side started to come loose. The lack of stability in the screws caused an imbalance in the function of the stool by disrupting the alignment of the hinge on the opposite side, which ultimately led to its demise. I should have just tightened those darn screws...

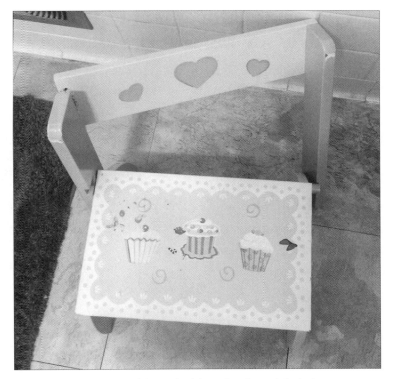

Figure 3.2 The loose hinges in this potty step relate to how dysfunctional joints in the body can affect others.

"Don't add strength to dysfunction."
—*Gray Cook*

The joint-by-joint approach to functional strength training should provide an easy-to-follow guide to improving physical performance and longevity for all populations. Quite simply, we should train mobile joints to become more mobile, and we should train stable joints to become more stable.

Keys to improving joint mobility
- Use consistent, comprehensive, joint-by-joint mobility and stretching movements
- Execute functional, multijoint exercises through a full range of motion

Keys to improving joint stability
- Improve strength in functional, multijoint patterns
- Prioritize unilateral exercises and free-weight training
- Emphasize deceleration and proper landing mechanics during jump training
- Refrain from exercises or movements that force stable joints to become more mobile (example: scorpion stretch with lumbar spine rotation)

Functional Movement Patterns Versus Muscle Groups

The body rarely uses one joint at a time to perform real-world movements and activities. With the exception of isolation-based strength training exercises and maybe your thumb clicking the TV remote, single-joint actions in the real world are few and far between when compared to the endless daily activities that simultaneously coordinate multiple muscle groups. These compound multijoint movements are often placed into categories called functional movement patterns. Although professionals in the movement and fitness fields offer slight variations as to how they categorize these patterns, most include some version of the movement categories listed below:

Functional movement patterns
- Knee-dominant
  - Squat
  - Lunge
- Hip hinge
- Upper body push
  - Horizontal push
  - Vertical push
- Upper body pull
  - Horizontal pull
  - Vertical pull
- Torso rotation
- Core stability*
  - Anti-extension
  - Anti-flexion
  - Anti-rotation
  - Anti–lateral flexion

*Although core stability consists of "anti" movements, a strong and stable core in all planes will improve efficiency in other compound functional movements.

A quality functional workout or training program should include a comprehensive balance of exercises from each category of movement patterns. Although there are some benefits to isolation-based strength training, such as targeted hypertrophy and joint-specific rehabilitation, these types of exercises should be prescribed *in addition to* functional movements, if at all. Each major muscle group will be used when all movement patterns are targeted in a training program. On the flip side, if each major muscle group is isolated in a training program, some movement patterns will be missed. Training-movement patterns should be the protein and potatoes of a functional strength training program, and isolation exercises should be the gravy.

Planes of Motion

Another key characteristic of functional strength training is that exercises are performed in all planes of motion. Although most traditional strength training exercises move in straight lines (usually up and down or forward and backward), there is so much more to how the body moves in the wild. If we only moved in straight lines, the world would look like a big game of Pac-Man. Instead, the body moves in three primary planes of motion (figure 3.3).

- Sagittal: Forward and backward, or up and down
- Frontal: Side to side, or lateral
- Transverse: Rotational

To maximize the benefits of a functional strength training program, exercises from each plane of motion should be incorporated at some level.

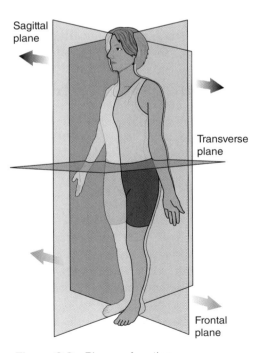

Figure 3.3 Planes of motion.

Although most functional strength training exercises take place in the sagittal plane, it is important to address the frontal and transverse planes regularly to prepare the body for the demands of daily activities and sports. See table 3.1 for exercise variation examples in each plane of motion.

Table 3.1 **Exercise Examples in Different Planes of Motion**

Primary pattern	Sagittal plane	Frontal plane	Transverse plane
Lunge	Forward lunge	Lateral lunge	Transverse lunge
Trunk movements	Straight leg sit-up	Kettlebell windmill	Medicine ball rotational throw
Bilateral jump	Box jump	Lateral box jump	Rotational box jump
Unilateral jump or leap	Split jump	Lateral leap	Rotational leap
Core stability*	Plank	Side plank	Anti-rotation hold
Upper body push or pull	Most upper body exercises are performed in the sagittal plane		

*A strong and stable core in all planes will improve efficiency in other compound functional movements.

We will address how to incorporate exercises from all planes of motion in later chapters when we discuss progressions, regressions, and program design. For now, the major takeaway is that you must select exercises from all planes of motion at some point to prepare the body for real-world demands.

Unilateral Versus Bilateral Exercises

When it comes to controversial topics among strength and conditioning coaches, religion and politics aren't in the same league as the discussion about unilateral versus bilateral exercise. (Although I'm being dramatic, some of the most decorated strength and conditioning coaches in the history of the field have conflicting opinions on this matter, and both sides have great points to support their stance.)

Unilateral exercises refer to movements that use a single leg or arm as the primary working limb, while bilateral exercises use both arms or legs equally. The controversy between these two camps usually surrounds unilateral versus bilateral lower body exercises.

To squat or not to squat? This controversy was sparked when Mike Boyle discussed what was dubbed as the "death of squatting" in his *Functional Strength Coach 3.0* DVD series released in 2009. Coach Boyle made it very clear that his advanced athletes no longer perform the conventional bilateral squat due to potential risks at heavy loads. Although he said nothing about the pros and cons of performing the bilateral squat as a fundamental compound movement at submaximal intensities, his comments provided fuel for a long-standing argument in our field that is still alive and well today.

Here are some of the main arguments that those on both sides of the discussion swear by:

Unilateral lower body exercises (figure 3.4)
- are more realistic or functional in nature because most daily activities and athletic movements are performed on one leg;
- require more coordination, proprioception, and stability, which will further reduce the risk of injury and improve performance; and
- are safer because an exercise can be performed at maximal intensity with much less weight, which reduces overall stress to the body, especially on the lower back.

Bilateral lower body exercises (figure 3.5)
- are fundamental compound movements that are key to building a solid foundation of strength and durability;
- require significantly more total load at maximal intensities, resulting in increased hormonal responses; and
- allow people to train at maximal intensities, which will elicit adaptations to the overall system, resulting in improvements to single-leg performance in training, sports, and daily life.

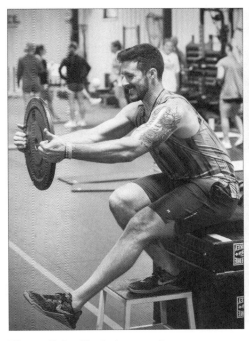

Figure 3.4 Single-leg squat.
Harife Gondogdu

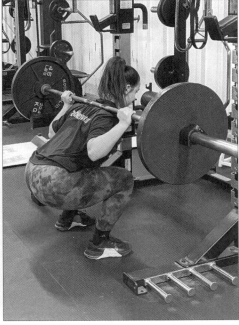

Figure 3.5 Back squat.

This book is dedicated to functional strength training in the physical education setting, and I believe it's important to expose students to both bilateral and unilateral exercises. Not only are bilateral exercises key early progressions in lower body functional movement patterns, but many ego-driven adolescents are going to squat and deadlift heavy weights no matter what. We might as well teach them the benefits of each approach and how to execute these skills correctly.

Debunking Common Strength Training Myths

Despite the availability of instant information at our fingertips, fitness myths are more common than one would think. These myths are often fueled by the onslaught of overnight fitness gurus and constant "magic pill" fads that flood our online media channels. Although you would hope students could rely on their PE teachers to sift through the garbage and provide only the facts, this is not always the case.

This section discusses some of the most common misconceptions I have heard over the years. It's important to air out these myths to provide PE teachers with factual information they can use to point their students in the right direction toward their fitness goals.

Spot Training

The number of times people have asked me what exercises they can do to get rid of the fat in a particular area of their body is staggering. The old myth that fat turns into muscle is completely false (Davidson 2021). There is no such thing as targeting a specific place on your body to magically get rid of the fat in that area. Is it possible to build muscle in specific locations to increase lean mass? Yes, but that does not mean the fat in that area is going anywhere. The only way to lose fat is to live in a consistent calorie deficit, as previously mentioned. Genetic predisposition and body type will determine where fat will shed first and where common trouble areas will linger. One of Mike Boyle's best dad jokes to date is that the best exercise for a six-pack is *table pushaways*. Ba-dum-ching! A six-pack comes from changing your overall body composition by focusing on nutrition first, not by crushing hundreds of crunches a day. Everyone already has a six-pack in there somewhere.

The Harder the Workout, the Better

The difficulty of an exercise or workout should not determine its effectiveness. Quality movement, appropriate intensity and volume, and progressive overload should be what defines a good day at the gym. The old-school mentality that glorifies soreness and crawling to the finish line of a workout is a turnoff for many who just want to feel, look, and perform better. Although pushing through physical stress and experiencing mild soreness can be common byproducts of a strength training program, a workout should not be frowned upon if participants are able to walk out of the gym under their own power.

At the peak of CrossFit's popularity, many affiliates would use unofficial mascots known as "Uncle Rhabdo" (as in *rhabdomyolysis*, which is a serious condition caused by overtraining that can lead to death or permanent damage) and "Pukie the Clown" to place a badge of honor on physical pain experienced during workouts. Although CrossFit's participation exploded during this time, I wonder how many people ran for the hills instead of picking up a free weight after seeing these images? I am sure most new-age CrossFit owners and corporate executives cringe at the thought of these mascots today, but it goes to show how the mentality of some hard-core fitness enthusiasts may influence the perception of strength training for the general public.

Squats Are Bad for Your Knees and Deadlifts Are Bad for Your Back

Bad squats are bad for your knees and *bad* deadlifts are bad for your back. However, performing these exercises with proper form, intensity, and volume can drastically improve the function and durability of these areas. Unfortunately, many people perform squats and deadlifts with improper technique and far too much weight, which can lead to serious injury and ongoing horror stories surrounding these normally harmless fundamental movements. This is why it is so important to introduce proper form and safe training methods to people of all ages.

When I started teaching physical education at Victor Central Schools in New York, there were stories of a medical doctor who met with our staff before I worked there, lobbying to ban squats and deadlifts from PE classes and athletics due to the potential dangers. Fortunately, our athletic director and PE staff members understood the importance of these movements, when performed correctly, for physical wellness and performance and were hesitant to take this advice. It's a shame that some medical professionals continue to steer people away from these beneficial exercises due to outdated misconceptions. During a Certified Functional Strength Coach course we hosted at Next Level Strength and Conditioning several years back, well-known strength coach and instructor Marco Sanchez put it perfectly when discussing this topic. He said, "If your physical therapist doesn't deadlift, it's time to find a new PT." Fortunately for us, our partnered physical therapist at Next Level, Dr. Russ Manalastas with MANA Performance Therapy, prescribes the deadlift for himself and clients of all shapes and sizes as much as my dentist recommends floss.

Strength Training Will Make Females Big and Bulky

Another outdated misconception is that females and males should train differently. Until fairly recently, a common thought process was that females should not strength train like males because they will develop unwanted muscle mass, resulting in masculine features and decreased flexibility. The good news is that the narrative has changed within the strength and conditioning field and popular culture in recent years, leading to more females participating in strength training programs that are on a level playing field with those of their male counterparts. The bad news is that many females still shy away from strength training because they believe they will end up looking like a muscle-bound beast if they step foot in a weight room. One of the biggest challenges when working with females is convincing them that strength training is both beneficial and necessary, regardless of gender, and that there is no reason to fear these unwanted results.

When speaking with females who may be hesitant to start strength training, it's important to stress that there are drastic differences in hormone levels between females and males. Elevated testosterone levels allow adolescent and adult males to gain muscle mass much more easily than females when consistently participating in a strength training program (Handelsman et al. 2018). Although females may notice a slight increase in muscle mass after several weeks of consistent strength training, it will not compare to the increases most males will experience from a similar training regimen. In addition, functional strength training can increase flexibility and mobility if performed through a full range of motion, as previously mentioned.

I have worked with many females who have visions of bodybuilders flexing on the stage when they voice their reservations about starting to strength train. Female bodybuilding is one of the most impressive sports on the planet due to the amount of dedication required for a female to build that much muscle despite naturally lower testosterone levels, and to prove this to hesitant females, I use examples of well-known celebrities and athletes who strength train consistently but do not look like competitive bodybuilders. One of my go-to examples of a strong female who strength trains regularly is swimsuit model and actress Kate Upton (figure 3.6). Anyone who follows Upton's personal trainer, Ben Bruno, on social media has seen videos of Upton performing a wide range of functional strength training exercises with an impressive amount of weight. I think it's safe to say that she has not developed an excessive increase in muscle mass while participating in functional strength training workouts over the past several years. If anything, Upton and Bruno have started a movement that has changed how many females view the benefits of strength training and false myths surrounding the topic. Not only has Bruno compiled a long client list of famous actresses and models in the process, but he has become a regular on many popular television shows preaching the value of functional strength training for women.

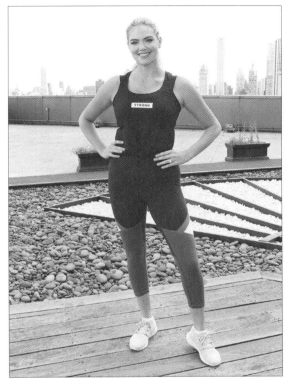

Figure 3.6 Kate Upton.
Cindy Ord/Getty Images

What's Next

The next chapter will discuss exercise selection using progressions and regressions as the cornerstone. There are countless "great" exercises out there, but it is important to select appropriate movements that serve a specific purpose to maximize results and safety.

4

Functional Strength Training Progressions and Regressions

Skill progressions are the building blocks of all sports, recreational activities, and strength training programs. Regardless of the activity, related skills tend to range from basic to complex, which provides a sequential road map that can be used to optimize the skill development process. This is common sense in many other areas of life:

- Roll → crawl → stand → walk → run
- Foundation → framing → drywall → paint → furniture
- Addition → subtraction → multiplication → division → whatever comes next

Join a gym and bang out 30 barbell snatches and 100 burpees for time on day one? No.

Although a sequential approach seems like common sense, when applied to fitness and strength training, people often skip steps, which can lead to injury, stunted results, and frustration. Quality physical education units are designed using sequential skill progressions as the foundation, so this thought process is second nature for most PE teachers. Good teachers would never introduce the layup before dribbling or the butterfly stroke before the front crawl. Fundamental principles should also be at the forefront of the functional strength training program, curricula, and lesson planning process.

Implementing Skill Progressions and Regressions

When applied to functional strength training, I would summarize the implementation of skill progressions and regressions as follows:

- A sequential list of exercises for each movement pattern or performance focus that puts variations in order by complexity, providing meaningful guidance during exercise selection in an effort to optimize physical development and safety.
    - Skill progressions increase complexity (basic → advanced)
    - Skill regressions decrease complexity (advanced → basic)
    - Skill lateralizations have a similar level of complexity but a different plane of motion, use of implements, or other potential factors

Functional skill progressions and regressions can be used as follows to optimize development and safety.

- Use sequential skill variation lists as a road map for programming, curriculum design, and lesson planning.
    - Pick exercises from each movement pattern and performance focus to develop a comprehensive fitness program or workout.
    - When in a group or class setting, start with variations that are appropriate for most participants based on ability and experience.
    - Increase complexity as participants master previously introduced skill variations.
- Use sequential skill variation lists to provide individualized modifications.
    - Select skill variations *before* training sessions, based on individualized needs and goals. Regress or lateralize skill variations for individuals in the group setting in advance if they are unable to perform an exercise due to ability, experience, or physical limitations.
    - Use skill regressions and lateralizations *on the fly* during a training session or class if an individual is unable to perform a skill correctly, despite additional cueing and slight modifications.

Example Skill Variations

Countless skill variations can be considered for each movement pattern and performance focus category. Fitness professionals may have slight differences of opinion based on their experience and general philosophies, because skill variation lists can be quite subjective. In addition, these lists often evolve over time based on trial and error, logistics, and the discovery or creation of new exercise variations. For the purposes of this book, which focuses on the PE setting, we will stick with the fundamental variations for each focus category. Tables 4.1 to 4.11 present variation lists for each movement pattern and performance focus. Lateralizations, where listed, are used in addition to, not in place of, the primary skill variation.

By no means are the variation lists in tables 4.1 to 4.11 set in stone or the only acceptable order of exercises, but I can justify the skill progressions based on years of personal experience in the physical education and sport performance settings.

Table 4.1 Knee-Dominant Exercises (Squats and Lunges)

	Primary skill variation	Lateralization
BASIC	Free squat (body weight)	*Step-up*
	Goblet squat	*Back lunge*
	Front squat or back squat	*Forward lunge*
	Split squat	*Lateral squat*
	Rear foot elevated split squat	*Lateral lunge*
COMPLEX	Single-leg squat	*Transverse lunge*

Table 4.2 Hip Hinge

	Primary skill variation	Lateralization
BASIC	PVC hinge and PVC RDL	
	Kettlebell deadlift	
	Hex bar deadlift	
	Loaded RDL	*Bilateral Slideboard leg curl*
	Single-leg RDL	*Single-leg hip lift (elevated back)*
COMPLEX	Skater squat (single-leg deadlift)	*Single-leg Slideboard leg curl*

Abbreviation: RDL = Romanian deadlift.

Table 4.3 Upper Body Push (Horizontal)

	Primary skill variation	Lateralization
BASIC	Push-up (elevated hands → hands on floor)	
	Barbell bench press	
	Dumbbell bench press	*Incline dumbbell bench press*
	Alternating dumbbell bench press	*Alternating incline dumbbell bench press*
COMPLEX	1-Arm dumbbell bench press	*1-Arm incline dumbbell bench press*

Table 4.4 **Upper Body Push (Vertical)**

	Primary skill variation	Lateralization
BASIC	Half-kneeling 1-arm kettlebell or dumbbell press	*Half-kneeling landmine press*
↓	Standing alternating kettlebell or dumbbell press	*Standing landmine press*
	Standing 1-arm kettlebell or dumbbell press	*Staggered-stance landmine press*
	Staggered-stance 1-arm kettlebell or dumbbell press	*Landmine push-press*
COMPLEX	1-Arm kettlebell or dumbbell push–press	

Table 4.5 **Upper Body Pull (Horizontal)**

	Primary skill variation	Lateralization
BASIC	TRX or barbell inverted row	*Half-kneeling cable 1-arm row*
↓	Standing 1-arm dumbbell or kettlebell row	*Standing cable 1-arm row*
	Kickstand 1-arm dumbbell or kettlebell row	*Staggered-stance cable 1-arm row*
	1-Arm TRX row	
COMPLEX	Bird dog 1-arm dumbbell or kettlebell row	

Table 4.6 **Upper Body Pull (Vertical)**

	Primary skill variation
BASIC	Tall kneeling cable or band pull-down
↓	Half-kneeling 1-arm cable or band pull-down
	Chin-up (palms in)
	Chin-up with neutral grip (palms facing each other)
COMPLEX	Pull-up (palms out)

Note: Lateralization does not apply.

Table 4.7 **Power**

	Primary skill variation	Lateralization
BASIC	Box jump	*Medicine ball chest pass*
↓	Squat jump	*Medicine ball shot put throw*
	Broad jump	*Medicine ball rotational throw*
	Split jump	*Lateral leap*
	Hang clean pull	*Hex bar or dumbbell jump with reset*
	Hang high pull	*Continuous hex bar or dumbbell jump*
COMPLEX	Hang power clean	

Table 4.8 Core Stability (Anti-extension)

	Primary skill variation
BASIC	Plank
↓	Stability ball rollout
	Wheel rollout
COMPLEX	Body saw

Note: Lateralization does not apply.

Table 4.9 Core Stability (Anti-flexion or Loaded Carry)

	Primary skill variation
BASIC	Farmer carry
↓	Goblet carry
	1-Kettlebell front rack carry
COMPLEX	1-Kettlebell overhead carry

Note: Lateralization does not apply.

Table 4.10 Core Stability (Anti-rotation)

	Primary skill variation	Lateralization
BASIC	Bird dog	
↓	Plank with alternating 1-arm reach	*Anti-rotation hold**
	Bear crawl	*Anti-rotation press**
COMPLEX	Lateral bear crawl	*Diagonal chop and lift**

*Tall kneeling → half-kneeling → in-line half-kneeling → standing → staggered stance.

Table 4.11 Core Stability (Anti–Lateral Flexion)

	Primary skill variation
BASIC	Side plank
↓	Staggered side plank
	Side plank with top leg elevated
COMPLEX	Suitcase carry

Note: Lateralization does not apply.

What's Next

Now that we have outlined how to properly select skill progressions that will allow people to safely and effectively achieve their personal fitness goals, the next chapter will discuss why functional strength training should be a priority in all physical education programs.

PART II

Functional Strength Training for Physical Education

In this section, I use nearly 20 years of experience in both the fitness and PE fields to tailor these overarching concepts to the classroom setting. Chapters 5 through 8 provide you with a comprehensive guide to curriculum design, teaching considerations, modifications for special populations, and assessment, specific to functional strength training in PE at all levels.

5

Why Functional Strength Training in Physical Education?

Fitness units are a staple in most K-12 PE programs. Lifetime physical fitness should be the cornerstone of a quality PE program's mission statement, so this makes sense. Most common fitness units introduce the benefits of physical activity, the five components of fitness, the frequency, intensity, type, and time (FITT) principle, and a wide range of movement options to choose from outside of school. Most of this information is very consistent because it's science driven, which doesn't allow much room for interpretation.

However, the application of concepts within PE fitness units can be very inconsistent, based on the experience and philosophy of the teachers designing the curriculum. Many programs focus primarily on cardiovascular activities, whereas others introduce basic strength training concepts and skills. Certain programs break down functional strength training skills into meaningful progressions, some use selectorized machines and isolation exercises, and others put students through boot camp–style workouts that are often far too complex. If the science surrounding fitness is so clear-cut and consistent, then why is there so much disparity between what students are exposed to in physical education? In most cases, it's because teachers like to teach what they know, what they enjoy, and what they're comfortable with.

To improve the quality and consistency of fitness units in the PE setting, teachers should focus on activities that will most benefit students if they choose to adopt those lifestyle habits outside of school. In reality, the only physical activity some students will receive may be during PE class, due to a drastic increase in average screen time. Regardless, the ultimate goal should be to inspire students to participate in daily physical activity outside of school and develop the skills and knowledge necessary to be successful independently.

Benefits of Functional Strength Training in Physical Education

Quality PE fitness units should incorporate all five components of fitness to provide a comprehensive experience (figure 5.1).

Functional strength training covers all these bases. Although there is plenty of room to introduce additional fitness activities such as distance running, biking, swimming, yoga, and more, implementing functional strength training in physical education by following a sequential road map will provide students with a safe, all-encompassing experience that can be applied to a lifetime of wellness.

Challenges of Implementing Functional Strength Training in Physical Education

Despite overwhelming evidence pointing to the benefits of implementing sequential functional strength training in PE units for students of all ages, it is often much easier said than done. Most teachers do not operate in their

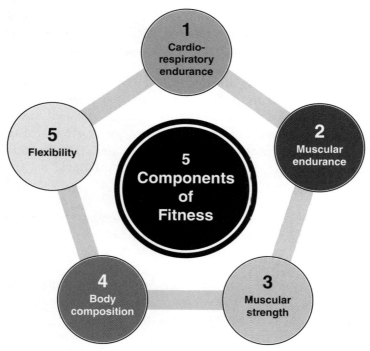

Figure 5.1 Five components of fitness.

own silo, so making significant program changes requires several people in a building or districtwide department to agree and work together. Unfortunately, people who are not willing to devote the time and effort necessary to implement changes are the biggest hurdle in adopting new concepts such as functional strength training in physical education. Although our profession is full of driven, dedicated, and progressive teachers who are willing to do whatever it takes to provide a meaningful experience for students, there are still plenty of stereotypical old-school "gym teachers" out there, just waiting to collect their pensions.

While giving presentations on functional strength training in physical education to countless teachers over the past several years, I have heard every excuse in the book, particularly from those who would rather just stick to traditional, machine-based fitness units. Change can be difficult, and it often requires a great deal of extra effort; therefore, much of the hesitation is valid. However, some stubborn teachers dig their heels in and refuse to consider change, perhaps out of pure laziness and lack of pride in our profession. Regardless of the situation, passionate teachers who are driven to implement functional strength training in physical education must find a way to get as many people on board as possible.

Here are some of the most common excuses and reasons for hesitating that I have heard over the years. Having an answer or possible solution to these in advance can help break down barriers when speaking to teachers who may be on the fence.

"If it isn't broken, don't fix it. This is what we've always done." It is our job as physical educators to always be on the lookout for the latest and greatest activities to offer our students. Teachers should have enough pride in our profession to change with the times and offer cutting-edge programming that will have the greatest possible benefits for students into adulthood. Earn your paycheck.

Teachers may need to learn new skills and concepts. Learning new skills and concepts takes additional time and effort, but again, it's what our students deserve. With adequate guidance and resources, it will be much less work than most people think.

Teachers may need to demonstrate skills they are uncomfortable with or may not be able to perform due to physical limitations. This excuse has been the biggest hurdle I have faced over the years. People like to teach activities they are comfortable with. When teachers are not confident in their own ability to demonstrate functional skills due to physical limitations or a lack of previous exposure, they tend to put up a massive wall. The good news is that teachers do *not* need to demonstrate these exercises in class! Teachers can use video demonstrations (see HK*Propel* for examples) and ask highly skilled students to demonstrate for them. This has been a game changer for teachers who have put up roadblocks due to their own insecurities.

Districts have limited budgets and space for physical education. Functional strength training requires a fraction of the space and money that traditional fitness machine units do. As we will discuss in later chapters, all you need to teach quality functional strength training units is some open space and a few free weights. No bells and whistles are necessary.

Teachers think they need to be a certified strength and conditioning coach or personal trainer to teach functional strength training. Functional strength training units in physical education should focus on fundamental skill development and basic fitness concepts. With the step-by-step road map and accompanying resources in this book, any qualified PE teacher can present this type of training safely and effectively to students. Certified strength and conditioning coaches and personal trainers apply these skills and concepts to specific personalized goals and needs at a more complex level than should be introduced in the general PE setting.

Teachers think that teaching functional skills will require more classroom and behavior management. I have actually found that the opposite is true. In my experience, I have been able to keep students more engaged and motivated by teaching them these fun, exciting, and self-fulfilling functional skills compared to traditional machine-based circuits. I believe students are much more likely to misbehave if they are given a list of machine exercises to complete on their own over a period of time, without any feedback or introduction of new skills.

Teachers, athletic directors, and PE directors do not want to waste money they spent on selectorized machines. Selectorized machines not only provide fewer benefits than functional exercises, but they take up a lot of valuable space and are extremely expensive compared to free weights. Therefore, when department leaders ask me how to improve their teaching space to implement functional strength training, I usually start with suggesting they get rid of most of their selectorized machines. People usually have a very hard time parting ways with several thousand dollars' worth of equipment, regardless of the situation. We will discuss facility design and equipment needs in later chapters, but except for a few machines that target functional patterns for populations with special needs and for elderly community members, I believe this equipment is a waste of space. Some options to get rid of selectorized machines without a total loss include buyback programs with equipment distributors, community yard sale events, and donating to local organizations for tax credit. The return will most likely be pennies on the dollar, but it's better than nothing.

Tips for Implementing Functional Strength Training

If you are reading this book, you are most likely passionate about implementing functional strength training in your current or future professional role. Although districtwide change requires a team effort, every department needs someone like you to take the lead. Here are some useful strategies that have worked for me in the past when trying to motivate hesitant teachers to give functional strength training in physical education a chance.

Start With Small Changes

Although you may want to give your program a complete overhaul right away, if you're dealing with difficult people and other potential hurdles, you may be better off making gradual changes to start. Once people see these changes in action, walls will start to break down, clearing a path to long-term change.

Know When to Bend

If a teacher who is putting up roadblocks feels strongly about keeping something in the program that you would like to remove, it may actually present an opportunity to gain trust and additional support. As long as it is safe for students, compromising in these situations can go a long way.

Speak Like a Coach

Many PE teachers also coach in the district. I have found that many of the teachers who resist change care more about their coaching position than their PE day job. Pointing out that functional strength training can drastically improve sport performance and decrease the risk of sport-related injury can be a huge selling point.

Gain Support from Athletic and PE Directors

Every district is different, but most top-notch PE programs have top-notch leaders at the helm. It is much easier to get everyone on board with change when it starts at the top. Start by selling the benefits of functional strength training to program leaders, then create a plan for districtwide implementation.

Realize That You Can't Win Them All

Unfortunately, no matter what you do, there may be people who flat out refuse to adopt these program changes. If you have done your part to help relieve hesitation without any success, you may need to move on without them. Although districtwide consistency is ideal, exposing some of your students to these concepts is at least a start. There is always the chance that reluctant teachers will slowly come around after seeing functional strength training in action.

What's Next

Now that we have discussed strategies to overcome common roadblocks that may cause some teachers to give up when implementing functional strength training in the PE setting, the next chapter will outline the curriculum design process to help teachers put these concepts into practice.

6

Curriculum Design

In a perfect world, all school districts would adopt a sequential curriculum for each PE unit to provide teachers with an easy-to-follow road map leading straight to PE Narnia, full of happy teachers working together to deliver life-altering experiences to their students. As we all know, perfection is not always possible. When giving presentations on functional strength training to current professionals over the years, the topic of curriculum design is where I have started to lose people who refused to believe that this fairy tale is achievable. In many cases, they are right. Based on their current situations, designing and implementing a working sequential curriculum is about as simple as advanced calculus. So before I go any further with curriculum design, please do not get discouraged if, at this point, your current situation will not allow for this level of planning and collaboration to come to fruition. If you start by slowly replacing machine-based isolation exercises with developmentally appropriate functional skills, you and your students are winning! On the flip side, you will be amazed at what you can accomplish with the right amount of effort and time. No matter what logistics stand in your way, designing and implementing a sequential curriculum can be a realistic long-term goal in most cases.

The Victor Way

Shortly after student teaching, I was fortunate enough to stumble into a nationally decorated PE program at Victor Central Schools in western New York. Although people talk a big game in college about what the perfect PE program should look like, I thought it was all very ambitious for the real world, based on my previous experiences. It wasn't long after starting at Victor that I realized they were actually walking the walk. Led by legendary athletic director Ron Whitcomb, I have never seen such a dedicated and passionate group of educators doing whatever it took to create life-changing experiences for their students. It was eye opening and inspiring. Not only were teachers exposing students to unique and progressive activities, but they had a working K-12 sequential curriculum in place with assessments at all levels. Of note, this is also where I start to see some eyes roll when I am presenting to current teachers. For the record, I am not trying to brag about how amazing Victor physical education is, and I am not suggesting that if you can't get to this level, you are failing. These systems were already in place when I got there, so I can't take credit for them. However, I can tell you that it is possible, and I have seen the benefits in action. It took years of trials and tribulations to create this standard for physical education in our district, but the hard work paid off in the end.

Benefits of a Sequential Curriculum

The benefits of having a step-by-step road map for each unit across the district was obvious to me from day one. For every unit, there was a working document outlining what primary skills needed to be introduced, assessed, and reviewed at each grade level. Instead of throwing darts at random topics during the unit-planning process, there was structured guidance to ensure students were being exposed to appropriate skills based on previous and future learning experiences. For me, this took all the guesswork out of planning. I knew what skills and concepts students had already been exposed to when they got to my class and what they would be exposed to at the next grade levels. My job was simply to connect the dots. Although teachers can plan amazing units without a sequential curriculum in place, they run the risk of either wasting time by teaching skills and concepts students have already mastered or leaving gaps that may impact long-term development. Unit planning without a continuum in place is kind of like planning a cross-country road trip without considering the geographic location of each city. New York City → Las Vegas → Chicago → Los Angeles→ Philadelphia? That seems like a lot of wasted gas money (figure 6.1).

One major misconception is that teachers must all teach everything exactly the same when following a curriculum. This is far from the truth. Teachers have the autonomy to plan their own unique units and lessons based on logistics and preferred activities. As long as students are exposed to the primary skills identified in the curriculum that will connect the dots from grade to grade, any variation in content delivery is fair game.

Design Down, Deliver Up

A term we use during the curriculum design process in Victor is *design down, deliver up* (figure 6.2). The first step in the process is to determine what you want students to know and be able to do in each unit by the time they graduate as seniors. Then, work backward from complex (final product) to basic (starting point), embedding skill progressions and concepts in reverse until you reach the ground floor. The design down, deliver up approach to curriculum will provide a solid sequential framework that teachers can use as a guideline to deliver grade-appropriate content

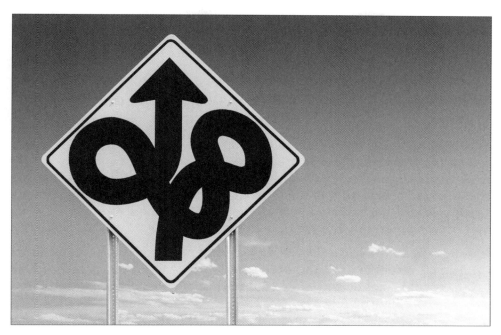

Figure 6.1 Lesson planning without a curriculum for guidance is like going on a road trip without considering the geographic locations of each stop.
ryasick/E+/Getty Images

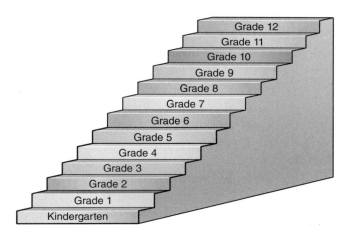

Figure 6.2 The design down, deliver up method.

throughout the student's educational experience, starting in kindergarten. I am no construction expert, but I assume builders start with a vision of what they want the skyscraper to look like and then work backward in the design process, instead of pouring the foundation first and designing the building floor by floor as they go.

For many units, including functional strength training, the first several floors of the building consist mainly of general gross motor skills and basic concepts that can be applied to multiple units in later years. However, these fundamental movement competencies are intentionally implemented to build a solid foundation for more advanced, unit-specific instruction to follow.

Enduring Understandings of Functional Strength Training

When using the design down, deliver up method to create a quality K-12 sequential framework in the area of functional strength training and fitness, we must start by determining what enduring understandings students should possess when they graduate from high school. For graduating seniors to successfully participate in comprehensive functional strength training and fitness programs into adulthood, they should

- believe in the *why*—that is, they should recognize the value of functional strength training and how it will help them achieve their personal goals so that they choose to adopt a comprehensive fitness plan on their own time;
- understand how to organize personal workouts by applying functional strength training skills to the frequency, intensity, type, and time (FITT) principle—to be successful on their own, they must know what exercises to select, how many sets and repetitions to perform, how much intensity to use, and how often they should participate in functional strength training workouts to reach their individualized goals;
- possess the skill proficiency necessary to perform functional strength exercises with proper form on their own in order to maximize results and safety;
- be able to identify local community resources where they can participate in functional strength training workouts independently or receive quality advanced training beyond their K-12 educational experience; and
- comprehend how cardiovascular exercise, sports, general physical activity, nutrition, and lifestyle complement functional strength training to create a comprehensive fitness plan.

Applying Skill Progressions to a Sequential K-12 Curriculum Map

When determining where functional strength training skills should fall on the sequential K-12 curriculum map, begin by listing exercise variations in order of complexity for each movement pattern and performance focus.

- Knee-dominant exercises
- Hip hinge

- Upper body push
- Upper body pull
- Power
- Core stability

The variation lists outlined in chapter 4 can be used to determine the skills that are appropriate to teach to most students at each grade level, starting with the most complex (design down). It is highly unlikely that every skill listed will make the final cut, so it's important to focus first on the primary skills required for the general student population to reach their goals. Logistics and the baseline ability level of most students involved will determine what the final curriculum map will look like for each district.

Secondary Versus Elementary Skill Development

The age at which students should start being exposed to structured functional strength training skill practice in physical education is often debated. Both physical and mental aspects of learning must be considered when determining what is developmentally appropriate for students. Although elementary-level students may be able to safely perform functional strength training progressions with structured sets and repetitions, teachers must contemplate the appropriate approach to maximize interest and engagement. Although unique grade structures between different districts may play a role, based on my experience, I believe it is appropriate to start implementing structured functional strength training skill practice sometime between fifth and seventh grade. To simplify, I suggest reserving formal functional strength exercise practice for the secondary level, which is usually sixth or seventh grade, as students enter middle school or junior high school. However, functional skills can be introduced informally at the elementary level within fun games, warm-ups, and stations.

Secondary PE Functional Strength Training Curriculum Outline

There are endless possibilities when it comes to selecting functional exercises during the process of designing a secondary curriculum map. In most cases, teachers must consider time constraints, class sizes, the baseline ability level of students, and much more. Due to these factors, it is highly unlikely that teachers will be able to introduce all of the functional exercises listed for each movement pattern and performance focus in chapter 4, leaving a lot of room for variation at the discretion of teachers based on their circumstances, experience, and personal preferences. As long as they are using meaningful progressions to select safe, developmentally appropriate skills, there are unlimited acceptable options.

Sample Curriculum Map for Grades 6 to 12

Table 6.1 provides an example of a functional strength training curriculum map for grades 6 to 12, including all four movement patterns, power, core, and important concepts for each grade level.

Table 6.1 **Sample Functional Strength Training Curriculum Map for Grades 6 to 12**

Grade	Knee-dominant	Hinge	Upper body push	Upper body pull	Power	Core	Concepts
12	RFESS	Skater squat	Landmine push-press	Pull-up, assisted*	Hang power clean	Body saw	Resources, program design
11	Lateral Squat	SLRDL	Standing 1-arm press	1-Arm TRX row	Hang high pull	Suitcase carry	Volume and intensity
10	Split squat	BB RDL	DB bench	Neutral chin-up, assisted*	Hang clean pull	Plank with 1-arm reach	Exercise selection
9	Front squat	SB leg curl	Standing landmine press	Standing 1-arm row	Hex jump and reset	SB roll-out	FITT principle
8	Goblet squat	Hex deadlift	BB bench	Chin-up, assisted*	Split jump	Side plank	5 Components of fitness and why FST
7	Free squat	KB deadlift	Half-kneeling press	TRX row	Broad jump	Bird dog	5 Components of fitness and why FST
6	Step-up	PVC hinge and RDL	Push-up with elevated hands*	BB inverted row	Box jump	Plank	5 Components of fitness and why FST
Added warm-up or station and workout options	Front and back lunges Lateral and transverse lunges	Snap-downs Hip lifts	Push-up variations Crawling	Arm slides Band or cable rows	Dynamic warm-up Ladders Hops, leaps, and jumps MB throws	Loaded carries Crawling	5 Components of fitness

Abbreviations: BB = barbell; DB = dumbbell; FITT = frequency, intensity, type, and time; FST = functional strength training; KB = kettlebell; MB = medicine ball; RDL = Romanian deadlift; RFESS = rear foot elevated split squat. SB = slideboard; SLRDL = single-leg Romanian deadlift.

*Regressed variation of the exercise.

This type of curriculum map can serve as a guide to teachers when planning units and lessons. How these skills are implemented within the classroom may look very different based on logistics. Ideally, teachers will have enough time to review skills from previous years and teach the new variations outlined for the current grade level. However, some districts have mixed grades in physical education, which can drastically change what a curriculum map will look like. Others have limited time for each unit due to facility use and other factors. Regardless, if teachers select skills from multiple movement patterns and performance categories and build on progressions from year to year, students will receive valuable instruction that can result in lifelong benefits.

Working Around Logistics

Sometimes, the perfect curriculum is not realistic due to factors that are out of the teacher's control. Instead of giving up because there are logistical roadblocks, teachers must push forward and do the best they can with the hand they are dealt. To ensure students are building on previously learned skills and concepts, keep in mind that some direction is better than none at all. When teachers are forced to jump over common hurdles that stand in the way of the perfect curriculum, they can refer to the following suggested action steps.

Lack of communication and buy-in from colleagues. As previously discussed, sometimes you just need to move on without the difficult people and push forward with the teachers who believe in the benefit of adopting a sequential curriculum.

Lack of time, space, or equipment to introduce as many skills and concepts as the teacher would like. In order to match the time, space, and equipment you have available, cut back the number of movement patterns and performance categories in the curriculum map. For example, focus on just the following categories:

- Lower body (knee dominant or hip hinge)
- Upper body (upper body push or upper body pull)
- Core

You should intentionally introduce power exercises such as jumps, hops, leaps, and ladder drills during warm-ups.

Combined grade levels in physical education. It is OK to repeat skills 2 or even 3 years in a row if necessary. I have never had a student who was *too* good at the deadlift or squat. This also provides an opportunity for older students to take the lead in helping to instruct and provide feedback to younger students, which is an advanced level of learning.

Table 6.2 shows an example of a curriculum map that has been modified due to logistical limitations.

Table 6.2 **Sample Modified Functional Strength Training Curriculum Map for Grades 6 to 12**

Grade	Lower body	Upper body	Core	Concepts	Power in warm-ups
11-12	Split squat	Landmine press	Suitcase carry	Resources, program design	Hops and leaps
9-10	Hex deadlift	TRX row	Side plank	FITT principle	Ladder drills
6-8	Goblet squat	Push-up	Plank	Why FST	Squat jump and broad jump

Abbreviations: FITT = frequency, intensity, type, and time; FST = functional strength training.

Review-Teach-Introduce

To maximize skill development and retention, it is important to review primary exercises from previous grades and introduce skills that will be the main focus in future years, if logistics allow. In my previous curriculum design experiences, we have used the terms *review*, *teach*, and *introduce* to signify when skills will work their way into a block plan and how much time to designate for each.

Review

At the beginning of a unit, review skills that were the primary focus of previous years in stations or during guided workouts. Have students recall previously learned skill cues when possible. Reviewed skills typically are not formally assessed.

Teach

Teach skills that are the primary focus for each grade level on the curriculum map to connect the dots from previous to future skill progressions. If teachers conduct skill assessments in physical education, some or all of the skills in this category can be formally assessed. Assessment will be discussed in more detail in chapter 8.

Introduce

If time allows, introduce skills that will be the central focus in future grades later in the unit. This brief exposure to more advanced skills may enhance upcoming learning. Introduced skills typically are not formally assessed.

Using a Curriculum Map to Build a Unit Plan

Consider the following points when using a curriculum map to build a unit plan:

- After creating a curriculum map that meets the specific needs of your students and your district's logistics, work horizontally across the current grade level to determine what primary skills will be taught. Refer to previous and future grades if time will allow for skills to be reviewed and introduced.
- Create a block plan by outlining skills and concepts over the course of a unit, from lesson to lesson. Block plans will be individualized based on the number of lessons dedicated to the unit, the duration of each class, and other logistical considerations. Teachers have the ability to create unique block plans to suit their personal preferences as long as primary skills from the curriculum map are prioritized to close the gap from grade to grade.
- Use the block plan as a guide to design comprehensive lesson plans using your district's preferred format. Modify and adapt, if necessary, as the unit progresses.

Sample Block Plan

Table 6.3 displays a sample block plan using the sequential curriculum map in table 6.1, based on the following logistical considerations.

- Ninth-grade class
- Sixty-minute classes
- Eight-day unit
- Adequate space and equipment for up to 30 students
- The following formally assessed skills:
  - Front squat
  - Standing landmine press
  - Standing one-arm row
  - Hex jump and reset
- All secondary teachers in the district are following a sequential curriculum map for grades 6 to 12 (see table 6.1)

Table 6.3 **Sample Ninth-Grade Functional Strength Training Block Plan**

Day 1	Day 2
Unit intro: grading, safety, resources Review: why FST Review (warm-up): free squat, snap-down and hinge, broad jump Review and practice: hex deadlift (R) Teach and practice: front squat (T), landmine press (T) Guided workout: include all skills discussed today and review additional skills previously learned	Review: grading, safety, resources, why FST Introduce FITT principle (frequency); discuss Review (warm-up): plank, push-up, split jump Review and practice front squat (T), landmine press (T) Teach and practice 1-arm row (T), hex jump and reset (T) Guided workout: include all skills discussed today and review additional skills previously learned

Day 3	Day 4
Review: grading, safety, resources, why FST Discuss FITT principle (intensity) Review (warm-up): bird dog, side plank, step-up Peer assessment stations • Front squat (T) • Standing landmine press (T) • 1-Arm row (T) • Hex jump and reset (T) • Slideboard leg curl (T) • Stability ball roll-out (T) • BB bench press (R) • Cardio (not peer assessed)	Review: grading, safety, resources, why FST, FITT principle Discuss FITT principle (type) Stations • Front squat and landmine press (practice self-assessment) • Front squat and landmine press (teacher assessment) • 1-Arm row (T) • Hex jump and reset (T) • Slideboard leg curl (T) • Stability ball roll-out (T) • TRX row (R) • Cardio

Day 5	Day 6
Discuss FITT principle (time) Stations • 1-Arm row and hex jump reset (practice self-assessment) • 1-Arm row and hex jump reset (teacher assessment) • Slideboard leg curl (T) • Stability ball roll-out (T) • Half-kneeling press (R) • Chin-up (R) • Box jump (R) • Cardio • Hand out QUIZ STUDY GUIDE	UNIT QUIZ Introduce and practice split squat (I), DB bench (I) Guided workout: include all skills discussed today and review additional skills previously learned

Day 7	Day 8
Introduce and practice BB RDL (I), neutral grip chin-up (I) Design a functional workout using the provided template and a list of previously discussed exercises with a partner Perform the program with a partner	Introduce and practice hang clean pull (I), plank with alternate arm reach (I) Design a functional workout using the provided template and a list of previously discussed exercises with a partner Perform the program with a partner Return quizzes

Abbreviations: BB = barbell; DB = dumbbell; FITT = frequency, intensity, type, and time; FST = functional strength training; I = introduce; R = review; RDL = Romanian deadlift; T = teach.

FUNdamentals of Functional Strength Training in Elementary Physical Education

As previously mentioned, teachers must consider what is developmentally appropriate both mentally and physically before deciding what to teach in a PE class. The old wives' tale stating that strength training can stunt the growth of children was disproven a long time ago. Research actually shows that developmentally appropriate strength training can have positive effects on physical development (Dahab and McCambridge 2009). However, pump the brakes before you start filling your elementary school gym with squat racks and barbells. As discussed in earlier chapters, strength is relative. Developmentally appropriate strength training for young children rarely requires any additional external load. Teachers must also consider the mental engagement of students. Although teaching a six-year-old to power clean can make for a cool Instagram post, holding the attention of a full class of elementary students while teaching complex strength training exercises seems far-fetched.

To maximize development, interest, and safety, the "FUNdamentals" of functional strength training should be introduced to elementary-aged children through fun games, challenges, relays, and obstacle courses focusing on movement and exploration. As students move into later elementary years, teachers can start to introduce skill cues for basic functional exercises in warm-ups and stations, but you will be amazed at what young children can figure out on their own if you can provide the right environment for exploration.

Jeremy Frisch is the owner and director of Achieve Performance Training in Clinton, Massachusetts. Frisch is well known for being at the forefront of long-term athletic development (LTAD) due to his open-ended approach to movement exploration with young children. Frisch's Twitter page (@JeremyFrisch) is a gold mine of amazing ideas for play-based LTAD activities. His videos may just look like kids racing, jumping, rolling, and flipping at first glance, but there is meaning behind all of it. Although these play-based activities and obstacle courses are intentionally designed to build the foundation for more structured training in later years, the kids don't always need to know that. Children will get more out of a fun atmosphere, friendly competition, and playful exploration.

USA Hockey has also done an amazing job prioritizing LTAD with its American Development Model (ADM). Although USA Hockey's ADM is specific to the long-term development of hockey players, this framework provides guidance that can be applied to any sport and to the PE setting. According to the USA Hockey ADM website, the eight stages of ADM focus on age-appropriate progressions that prioritize the development of physical literacy, mental engagement, and lifelong participation.

ADM's Eight Stages

- Active Start Stage (ages 6 and under, beginners)
- FUNdamentals, Play to Learn (ages 6 and under to 8 and under)
- Learn to Train (ages 10 and under to 12 and under)
- Training to Train (ages 14 and under to 16 and under)
- Learn to Compete (ages 18 and under)
- Train to Compete (ages 20 and under, National Collegiate Athletics Association)
- Train to Win (International)
- Hockey for Life

USA Hockey also uses the Windows of Trainability chart to highlight gender-specific developmental stages and optimal opportunities to improve specific facets of performance based on the ability to adapt at each stage (figure 6.3). Based on the Windows of Trainability (Balyi, Way, and Higgs 2013), speed and suppleness (flexibility) should be the primary targets of physical development with children of early elementary age. This can be accomplished through a wide range of play-based activities. Informally

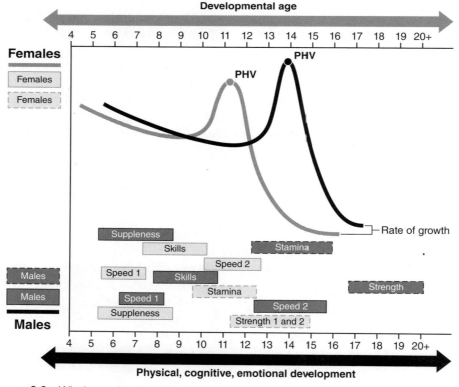

Figure 6.3 Windows of trainability.

introducing functional exercises and placing an emphasis on coordination in later elementary grades captures the "skills" window outlined below. I strongly suggest visiting USA Hockey's ADM website (www.admkids.com) to learn more.

The good news is that most elementary teachers already do an amazing job of creating fun and exciting opportunities for children to develop gross motor skills, speed, flexibility, and coordination within the PE setting. Although many of these suggestions for the building blocks of the functional strength training curriculum at the elementary level may seem open ended, there are some guidelines that will help build a strong foundation to support more complex skill development in secondary grades.

Elementary FUNdamentals of Functional Strength Training Objectives

- Introduce FUNdamentals of functional movement and performance within fun games and activities, with an emphasis on the following:
    - Sprinting and reactive change of direction
    - Flexibility
    - Body control and general coordination
    - Spatial awareness
    - Athletic posture
    - Core strength
    - Balance
    - Eccentric control and deceleration (landing, cutting, etc.)
    - Informal introduction to functional movement patterns
    - Character and leadership
- Create an exciting environment that will keep kids engaged and promote the value of physical fitness and movement
- Do no harm—consider and address safety concerns in advance

Elementary Functional Strength Progressions

Although I would not recommend introducing functional skill cues with structured sets and repetitions for children of early elementary age, implementing the general movements below in games, races, and obstacle courses can serve as early progressions for more complex exercises.

- Bear crawl → Push-ups
- Climbing → Pull-ups
- Changing levels/Climbing under objects → Squats/Lunges
- Changing levels/Climbing over objects → Hip extension
- Rolling → Core control
- Hanging → Loaded carries

- Jumping and Leaping from object to object → Hip hinge/Jumping/Leaping/Deceleration
- Balance beams → Single leg stability
- Medicine ball throws → Olympic lifts

Adapted from X, formerly known as Twitter, posts by Jeremy Frisch.

Obstacle Course Examples

Obstacle courses are a great way to incorporate a wide variety of developmentally appropriate functional movements in a fun, safe, and exploratory environment (figures 6.4 and 6.5). Here are some easy ways to incorporate elementary functional progressions in obstacle courses.

- Crawl under a low obstacle
- Hang or climb from point A to B (chin-up bars, traverse rock wall, ropes)
- Climb over big boxes or tall beams
- Climb under waist-high hurdles or ropes
- Roll from point A to B
- Jump to and from pads, mats, or objects on the floor (make sure these won't slip out from under people when landing)
- Walk across a balance beam
- Medicine ball slam or throw

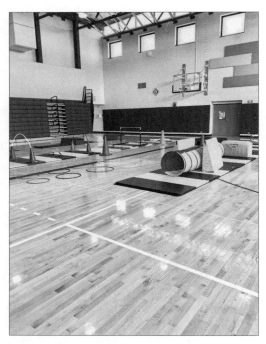

Figure 6.4 Physical education obstacle course at Victor Intermediate School (Victor, New York).

Chapter 6 • Curriculum Design   67

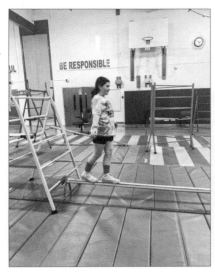
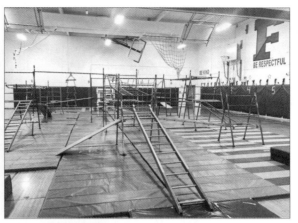
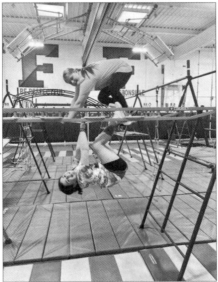

Figure 6.5 Physical education obstacle course at Northside Elementary (Fairport, New York).
Dennis McGurk

Elementary FUNdamentals Curriculum Map

There is much more open-ended guidance at the elementary level compared to the secondary curriculum map guidelines previously discussed. Teachers have the autonomy to expose elementary students to the FUNdamentals of functional strength training in an endless number of ways. If teachers follow the basic guidelines below, they are checking all of the boxes required to build a strong foundation for more structured skill development at the secondary level.

- Prioritize fun and friendly competition
- Make sure all activities are safe and developmentally appropriate
- Incorporate speed, change of direction, flexibility, and coordination daily

The elementary FUNdamentals curriculum map in table 6.4 outlines meaningful progressions and activity ideas for teachers to follow during the lesson planning process.

Table 6.4 **Elementary FUNdamentals Curriculum Map**

Grades	Speed and agility	Flexibility	Coordination	Strength
K-2	Tag games Relay races Obstacle courses	Expose students to a wide range of movements at different levels (over and under objects) and in a variety of planes of motion during obstacle courses and other games	Introduce gross motor skills including marching, galloping, skipping, lateral shuffling, and hopping	Incorporate elementary-level functional strength progressions previously listed within obstacle courses and other games
3-5	Tag games Relay races Obstacle courses Short sprints	Introduce basic stretching, mobility, and gymnastics	Introduce ladder drills, jump rope, and contralateral coordination exercises, including • Dead bugs • Bear crawls • Additional skipping variations	Introduce external skill cues to basic functional exercises in warm-ups and stations, including • Toe touch to squat • Snap-down and hinge • Plank • Elevated push-ups • Step-up • Inverted row

Connecting Functional Strength Training to National Standards

The 2024 SHAPE America National Physical Education Standards define what a student should know and be able to do as a result of a highly effective physical education program. States and local school districts across the country use the National Standards to develop or revise existing standards, frameworks, and curricula.

These standards provide teachers with specific targets that cover all bases necessary for students to receive a positive and comprehensive experience in the physical education setting. The ultimate goal of the standards is to provide the inspiration, skills, and knowledge required for students to achieve lifelong wellness.

2024 SHAPE America National Physical Education Standards

Standard 1: Develops a variety of motor skills.

Standard 2: Applies knowledge related to movement and fitness concepts.

Standard 3: Develops social skills through movement.

Standard 4: Develops personal skills, identifies personal benefits of movement, and chooses to engage in physical activity.

Reprinted by permission from SHAPE America, *National Physical Education Standards,* 4th ed. (Champaign, IL: Human Kinetics, in press).

What's Next

There are many teaching considerations that are unique to functional strength training and fitness units. The next chapter will outline several teaching strategies that will help teachers deliver meaningful instruction in this setting.

7

Teaching Considerations

Skill cues describe key components of a movement to provide students with the direction required to perform a skill correctly. Physical educators eat, breathe, and sleep skill cues. This is the primary vehicle for content delivery in the PE setting, so most PE teachers are skill-cue black belts. The best teachers in the field understand that not all skill cues are created equal. A good skill cue not only should result in the student performing a skill correctly but should make a deep connection, resulting in long-term retention. Internal and external skill cues are most commonly used when describing functional strength training and fitness exercises. Brendon Rearick does an excellent job of comparing internal and external skill cues in his book, *Coaching Rules* (2020). The definitions below are paraphrased from Rearick's coaching rule number 15.

Internal Skill Cues
- Direct attention to body parts and how to move
- Place attention on joints, muscle groups, angles of movement, and body position
    - Example (free squat): Keep your chest up and shoulders back

External Skill Cues
- Direct attention away from the body, focusing on the outcome of the movement in relation to the environment
- Use animated imagery, analogies, and descriptive action verbs related to the environment to make long-lasting connections
    - Example (free squat): Show off the logo on your shirt

Although there may be a time and place to use internal cues, studies have shown that external skill cues are more effective for learning, performance, and retention because they allow the motor system to self-organize with less conscious interference (Bartholomew 2023).

External skill cues are second nature to most PE teachers, especially with common units. These include *soldier-monkey-tree* (elementary backstroke), *high five and wave goodbye* (volleyball float serve), and *reach in the cookie jar* (basketball follow-through), to name just a few. However, for some reason, many teachers and coaches turn into wannabe kinesiologists when they start explaining fitness exercises. Not only are internal cues less effective than external cues for learning, performance, and retention, kids don't care how much you know about the body. If skill cues include muscle groups, joint angles, and other complex terms, they usually go in one ear and out the other.

Nick Winkelman is a master of external skill cues. Although he is a world-renowned sport performance coach, he uses external skill cues that some might even view as childish with his elite professional athletes. I used to rely on big scientific words, hard-to-pronounce muscles, and confusing joint angles when coaching my advanced athletes to prove that I knew my stuff. Coach Winkelman completely changed how I coach my college and professional athletes when I attended one of his seminars on external skill cues at a Perform Better summit several years ago. Experiencing the impact of Coach Winkelman's external skill cues during the hands-on portion of his workshop was a game changer for me. I will never forget some of the external cues he used, such as "balance a cup of tea on the knee" (figure 7.1) for an explosive knee drive with isometric hold and

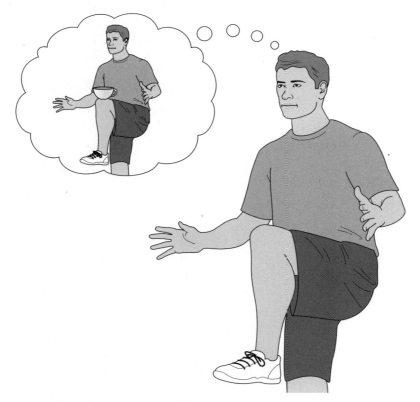

Figure 7.1 External skill cue example from Nick Winkelman: "Cup of tea on the knee."

so many more. He proved that not only do external cues result in better results and retention but that no one cares what fancy words you know. If one of the best sport performance coaches in the world could use these animated analogies with his professional rugby players, then why would I overcomplicate things to make myself feel like I was worthy? Since that time, I have used animated external skill cues whenever possible, regardless of the population's age or ability level, with a great deal of success.

Coach Winkelman's book, *The Language of Coaching* (2020), takes a deep dive into the art and science of teaching movement. I can't recommend this book enough for physical educators, fitness professionals, and sport coaches to enhance the impact of instruction. In his book, Winkelman uses the term *cueing in 3D* to maximize intent and direct focus toward the desired result. The three-dimensional concept breaks external skill cues into the following three subcategories.

1. Distance (example: close or far)
2. Direction (example: toward or away)
3. Description (action verb or analogy)

The ultimate goal is to incorporate all three subcategories within external skill cues whenever possible. Here is one example from *The Language of Coaching* (117).

Dumbbell Bench Press
- "Focus on smashing the dumbbells through the ceiling."
    - Description: smashing
    - Direction: through
    - Distance: ceiling

The appendix of this book has an extensive list of external skill cues for each functional strength training exercise that was listed in the secondary PE curriculum map in chapter 6. In addition, Winkelman's *The Language of Coaching* and Rearick's *Coaching Rules* are valuable treasure troves of amazing external skill cues. Rearick also created the website http://externalcues.com, where coaches and teachers can access his external skill cues and even contribute to the ever-growing list.

To take the value of external skill cues in physical education a step further, think about how beneficial it would be if students were exposed to consistent functional strength training cues across the district. Although there are countless quality external skill cues for every exercise, if department leaders can designate two or three cues that all teachers will use as baseline teaching points, student performance and retention will flourish. District strength and conditioning coaches can also join the party by coordinating with the PE department to adopt unified cues between physical education and athletics to further enhance skill development.

Class Management Strategies

Teaching functional strength training at the secondary level can present unique classroom management hurdles because the unit traditionally takes place in a weight room or fitness center, along with many other factors. The following strategies, based on my experience teaching functional strength training in the physical education and sport performance settings over the past several years, will help PE teachers navigate this environment and the potential challenges that may come with it.

Sell, Sell, Sell

As discussed in previous chapters, the more kids understand how functional strength training will benefit them in their daily lives, the more they will buy in during class and on their own time. Every day, revisit why functional strength training is so important for health, performance, and longevity. Speak "student" when introducing an exercise by relating the benefits of the exercise to what young people that age care about the most, which is usually performance in a wide variety of sports and activities, along with other short-term benefits previously mentioned.

Have Students Sit Down or Take a Knee During Instruction

Although this strategy can be beneficial for all units and settings, it is especially important in the weight room or fitness center due to the potential dangers in that environment. I have always said that *Saturday Night Live* should do a skit about what it's like teaching junior high students in a PE class. Any veteran middle-level teacher will tell you that if you let students stand during instruction, many will be walking in circles, busting out TikTok dances, poking their neighbor, or playing with something around them before you get your fifth word out. Having students sit or take a knee anchors them in one spot, which will improve focus and ensure all students can see your demonstrations.

Teach and Practice One New Skill at a Time

When introducing a skill for the first time, it is important to have students practice and receive feedback before moving on to the next exercise. During fitness units, some teachers introduce a multitude of new skills in stations or independent workouts before giving students the opportunity to practice, but by the time the teacher gets to the second or third exercise, most students will have forgotten the name of the first skill, let alone the important teaching cues. When teaching a new skill, follow the sequence below to maximize performance and retention.

- Describe the skill and the associated benefits.
- Demonstrate the skill using external cues.

- Have students practice; provide individual feedback.
- Revisit skill cues and points of emphasis with the class.
- Have students practice more, with individual feedback.

Once exercises have been introduced following this teaching sequence, they can be used in stations and independent workouts after a brief review of core external cues and a quality demonstration.

Organize Students in Straight Lines During Skill Practice

There are several benefits to designating predetermined practice areas set up in straight lines throughout the teaching space (figure 7.2). Organizing students in circles or allowing them to pick their own practice space in the room does not offer the same advantages for skill development and classroom management. Benefits to organizing students in straight lines include the following:

- Students look more organized, which can improve focus and help them stay on task during skill practice.
- Due to linear sightlines, it is easier for the teacher to observe students' form in a large group while they keep their "back against the wall." Teachers can scan down a line of students to quickly identify which students require feedback first, without losing sight of potential behavior or safety issues.
- Teachers can ensure that students will have enough personal space to practice skills safely and can methodically place students at ideal practice locations to avoid potential behavior problems if needed.

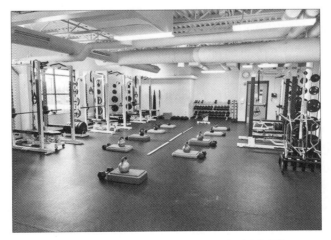

Figure 7.2 A Victor Central Schools junior high PE functional strength training lesson set up in straight lines.

Focus on Form First

Many adolescents (especially teenage boys) care more about how they compare to their peers than about performing skills with proper form. When students have the ability to choose their own weights during skill practice, the weights usually end up being far too heavy, which leads to poor form. "Use less weight" can be one of the most effective pieces of corrective feedback a teenager can receive when form starts to suffer. Although meaningful progressive overload is the golden goose of functional strength training, poor form due to excessive load can lead to bad habits and serious injury.

When introducing a new skill, keep the weight light so students can focus on form first. I suggest designating a submaximal intensity at each practice area that will allow all students in the class to perform the exercise with proper form when the focus is skill development. As students perfect their technique, teachers can begin to guide progressive overload on an individual basis, eventually allowing students to select their own weights during functional strength training workouts.

Lesson Sequencing

Lesson sequencing at the secondary level will be affected by many factors, including class duration, the lesson number in the unit, previous exposure to skills, and more. Although these factors may lead to a wide range of acceptable variations, the following is an example of a quality functional strength training lesson outline.

- Lesson introduction
    - Learning target and lesson objectives
    - Why, how, and what
        - Explain why the objectives in all three domains of learning are important and the benefits of the lesson's focus
        - Discuss how to achieve objectives and apply the lesson's focus outside of school
        - Describe what the lesson will entail (the daily agenda)
    - Review of important information from previous classes
- Warm-up or review activity
- Structured skill practice
    - Review previous skills
    - Teach new skills
- Apply new and reviewed skills in a guided workout or in stations
- Closure

- Check for understanding
  - Think-pair-share discussion
  - Self-assessment
- Overview of upcoming lessons

Safety Considerations

The number one priority of PE teachers should be to do no harm, regardless of the unit. It is critical that teachers consider potential safety hazards in advance and plan accordingly. Regularly addressing possible dangers related to the environment, etiquette, and behavior will help students stay safe during class and on their own time. The fitness center and weight room present unique opportunities for injuries to occur, which requires teachers to place an extra emphasis on the topic of safety. Here are some ways for physical educators to address the most common safety concerns related to functional strength training in this setting.

- Adjust the environment
  - Be sure that all equipment is in safe working order
  - Organize the space to allow for a safe flow of students
- Select developmentally appropriate exercises
  - Follow meaningful progressions that allow students to build on previously mastered skills
- Prioritize proper form
  - Make sure students can demonstrate perfect technique before adding external load
  - Modify exercises if students are unable to perform skills correctly due to ability level or individual limitations
- Prescribe an appropriate volume
  - Use general volume guidelines outlined in later chapters to target desired adaptations without the risk of overuse injuries
  - Understand that allowing students to perform exercises to the point of muscle failure presents significant safety risks
- Address spatial awareness
  - Students must always be aware of their surroundings to avoid contact with heavy objects, unforgiving edges, and other dangerous objects in this environment
- Incorporate spotting
  - To avoid obvious risks, spotters should be mandatory while performing the barbell bench press, regardless of the intensity; preach

the importance of quality spotting technique from the start to build good habits
- Spotting for exercises such as the deadlift and power clean should be prohibited due to the potential dangers to both parties
- Although spotting for the bilateral squat is common in the sport of powerlifting, I recommend teaching students to use power rack safety arms in place of a spotter in the PE setting
- Emphasize weight room and fitness center etiquette
    - Double check that the amount of weight on the barbell is accurate and secured with clips prior to each set
    - Return all equipment where it belongs at the completion of the final set, not at the end of the class or workout
    - Disinfect equipment after use
- Avoid burpees
    - Burpees are often prescribed in high volume for conditioning purposes, which can lead to sloppy variations of the exercise that resemble the worst "worm dance" you've ever seen; although it can be argued that each segment of the burpee, if performed with proper technique, is functional and beneficial, when performed as one exercise at high volumes with broken form, the risk of injury is not worth the benefit (Google search *Ben Bruno burpees* to learn more about why PE teachers should avoid this popular exercise with students)
- Prioritize daily movement preparation
    - Create good habits by incorporating a comprehensive movement preparation at the beginning of each class and stressing the benefits of injury reduction and performance enhancement to build buy-in (more details on movement preparation will be discussed later)

Functional Strength Training and the Affective Domain

The affective domain has always been a beneficial byproduct of quality physical education due to the elements of sportsmanship, teamwork, and cooperation associated with physical activity and sports. According to a recent article, "Affective Learning in Physical Education: A Systematic Review," teachers have the ability to make a greater impact on the mental and emotional health of students by intentionally targeting the affective domain in physical education (Teraoka et al. 2020). Planning outcomes directly related to the affective domain prior to instruction has been termed "pedagogies of affect." With the recent uptick in mental and emotional health concerns that children and teenagers are facing all over the world, PE teachers have the ability to influence the lives of students well beyond their physical health.

Functional strength training and fitness units present a unique opportunity for teachers to intentionally address important issues such as body image, self-esteem, anxiety, and depression due to the proven benefits connected to these issues (Gordon et al. 2020). With the inclusion of social-emotional learning (SEL) in schools, the direct connection between functional strength training and the affective domain in physical education is a good fit for the SEL narrative outlined in figure 7.3.

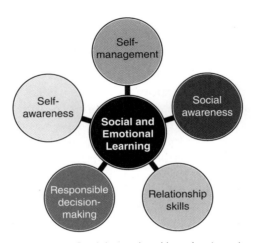

Figure 7.3 Social-emotional learning targets.

Modifications for Students With Disabilities

Students with special needs require strength for general health, performance in daily activities, and long-term durability, just like their peers. Unique daily challenges that many other students do not need to deal with can present additional needs for strength in order to combat the physical demands that come with certain disabilities. Unfortunately, students with significant needs often receive a modified PE curriculum that does not include strength training, because teachers do not know how to modify exercises or they are afraid of causing injury. In most situations, students can participate in some form of strength training safely, regardless of their situations.

Because there is a wide spectrum of cognitive and physical disabilities, concrete suggestions will not apply to all students. Modifications will depend on the unique, individualized needs of each student. Teachers will need to use their best judgment on a case-by-case basis to ensure that all students receive modified instruction that is safe and effective.

Regardless of the situation, teachers must prioritize safety. Always err on the side of caution, but this does not mean to avoid strength training altogether. In most cases, regressing skill selection to basic movements for each functional pattern and performance focus will allow students to participate safely and successfully.

For more significant special needs, teachers may need to alter activities beyond regressing skill selection. If a student has use of only one limb, for example, teachers can modify exercises to a unilateral skill. Examples include the following:

- Front squat → one-leg squat to box
- Bench press → one-dumbbell bench press
- Chin-up → half-kneeling one-arm cable pull-down

Selectorized machines can also be great tools that allow students with significant special needs to strength train safely, because the machine guides the user through the movement and there is very little risk of injury. Machines also allow teachers or aides to offer additional physical assistance if needed. Although I preach that we need to send most selectorized machines to the junkyard, I do recommend that districts keep a few machines for special populations. To maximize benefits and limit the space needed, I suggest prioritizing one upper body pull machine (horizontal row or vertical pull-down), one upper body push machine (horizontal push or vertical press), and a leg press machine. Some companies also offer multiuse cable systems that are fairly compact.

Regardless of the modifications required, the goal is to have all students safely participate in some form of strength training regularly to experience benefits that can drastically improve their quality of life.

What's Next

Now that we have covered skill progressions and teaching considerations for functional strength training units at all levels, we can roll the final credits, right? Hold your horses. How will teachers know if they were able to successfully teach the skills and knowledge necessary for students to be successful on their own time? Assessment! The next chapter will discuss realistic assessment strategies to drive accountability for learning while providing teachers with meaningful feedback.

8

Assessment

Assessment in physical education can be a sore subject for teachers who are resistant to change, because they do not understand the value. There is a common misconception that assessment in physical education requires a significant amount of extra time, effort, and recordkeeping from teachers, when in reality, it can be built into any common lesson plan without drastically affecting activity time or teacher workload. The people who picture long lines of students waiting to be assessed by teachers in lab coats are way off.

For many decades, most feedback from PE class was based purely on behavior. If students were busy, happy, and behaved well in class, they were doing A-OK. Even when there were performance categories on progress reports or report cards, they were usually based on informal observation, not reliable assessments with rubrics or checklists connected to learning objectives. Although I would like to say that this laissez-faire approach to assessment is a thing of the past, many PE teachers are still in this boat today.

When speaking to teachers who are hesitant about assessment in physical education, it is usually due to their misconceptions and lack of experience in this area. Once they let their walls down long enough to hear why assessment in physical education is so important and what it really looks like in action, most change their tune quickly. If physical education is to be taken seriously and valued as much as other subjects, we need to hold ourselves to a higher standard. With the guidance provided in this chapter, I hope teachers who are on the fence will realize how easy and valuable assessment in physical education can be and how to apply these methods to a functional strength training curriculum.

Why Assess?

What if grading in math class were like old-school physical education? Show up on time, bring your pencil and calculator, pay attention, follow directions, work well with others, and earn a 100%. Sign me up for that! Although all these intangible factors are important, what do they have to do with math? You start with a 0% in math and other core subjects, not 100%. You earn your grade based on assessment scores directly connected to grade-specific performance objectives. If our goal is to teach students the skills and knowledge required to successfully participate in physical activity outside of school, then why would assessment be any different in physical education?

Benefits of Assessment in Physical Education

The following are some undeniable benefits to assessing student performance in physical education.

Hold students accountable for learning. Just like any other subject, if students know what the unit objectives are, how they will be assessed, and how the assessment will impact their grade or progress report, most will put forth their best effort to learn the skills and knowledge required to do well on the assessment. This may motivate some less-skilled students to put in extra work with a teacher or at home to develop the tools they need to be successful on their own time. Without some form of performance assessment, there is no reason for students to push themselves to develop the skills and knowledge required to participate successfully outside of school. Recess and physical education are two different things. Although participating in physical activity during class is a crucial component of physical education, students must also be held accountable for learning in this setting.

Provide students with feedback. Not all assessments are at the end of a unit for a grade. There are formal, informal, summative, and formative assessments in physical education. Regardless of the situation, all assessments should provide students with feedback that can be applied to future skill development sessions and independent activities. Quality assessments will provide students with much more than a score, telling them exactly what they did well and what they need to improve on to further enhance their abilities.

Provide the teacher with feedback. Learning objectives and associated assessments should be designed to meet the needs of most students at each grade level. Teachers may need to find creative ways to challenge top-tier students beyond the targets designated for the rest of their peers, while other students may require additional attention to meet the desired level of achievement. If assessments are appropriate for the majority of the population, these outliers should be few and far between. When teachers notice that an exorbitant number of students are outside of targeted benchmarks, it may be time to look in the mirror; in some cases, learning targets may not be appropriate for the population at hand if most students struggle with assessments or do not seem challenged enough. A wide range of assessment scores may also tell teachers that they need to consider making changes to future lesson plans and teaching strategies to help students achieve grade-level learning objectives.

Process Versus Product

Process-based assessments focus on the steps required to perform a skill or task correctly, while product-based assessments focus solely on the outcome. Some assessments strictly focus on the process or product of a task, while others may incorporate both.

- *Process.* The student is able to perform five push-ups (hands on the ground or elevated) with proper technique (3 of 3 skill cues from a checklist).
    - The focus is purely form, due to the student's ability to modify the exercise (elevate hands) if they are not strong enough to do five standard push-ups with their hands on the ground.
- *Product.* The student is able to perform five standard push-ups (hands on the ground).
    - The focus is purely the strength outcome of performing five standard push-ups (hands on the ground), with no emphasis on proper form.
- *Process and product.* The student is able to perform five standard push-ups (hands on the ground) with proper technique (3 of 3 skill cues from a checklist).
    - The focus is both process and product, because students must perform the skill with proper form but also need to be strong enough to complete five repetitions with their hands on the ground, which is a strength-based outcome.

Most PE units incorporate both process- and product-based assessments. The process of a skill or task is the foundation of success and should be the priority, but the end result or product should become more of a priority as students get closer to graduation. On the same trajectory, most skill assessments should be conducted in controlled settings (stations) with younger children, whereas more assessments should take place in authentic situations (game play and program design) as students get older to prepare them for independent activity as an adult (figure 8.1).

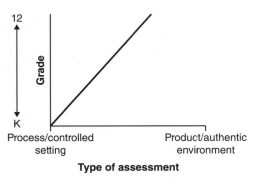

Figure 8.1 Process versus product.

I believe that fitness units should focus primarily on process-based objectives and assessments at all grade levels. Fitness and wellness are a personal, individualized, lifelong journey that requires a significant amount of dedication, time, and effort. Each person's journey will be different based on an endless list of factors, including starting point, fitness goals, genetics, skill level, motivation, and many more. Students should be focusing on their own fitness goals and personal progress instead of constantly comparing themselves to peers. Attempting to reach unrealistic outcome-based goals to keep up with others may lead to discouragement, obsessive behavior, and injury.

Process-based assessments in PE fitness units should focus on performing skills with proper technique, consistent participation in fitness activities, and healthy lifestyle habits. In my opinion, product-based fitness objectives that compare students' strength, endurance, speed, and body weight with those of their peers are not appropriate for the PE setting. Not all students are built the same, and that is OK. I believe making students feel inferior because they are unable to reach fitness benchmarks, regardless of their personal progress and effort, is counterproductive. However, regularly focusing on the benefits of fitness activities and consistent, healthy lifestyle habits as well as developing a wide range of fitness skills and the knowledge required to put it all in action will inevitably result in the residual product-based outcomes previously listed.

To Fitness Test, or Not to Fitness Test?

Fitness testing is another hot topic in the PE world. Based on my earlier statements supporting process-based objectives, assessments, and personal goals, I do not conduct fitness testing in the PE setting. Many amazing teachers may completely disagree with my stance on this topic, so the following are some reasons for my opinions.

Why do teachers conduct fitness testing in physical education? Most PE teachers will say that they conduct fitness testing to collect data that they can communicate with parents and use to create individualized fitness programs. Although this is great in theory, in my experience, it is rare to find teachers who are actually using the data to create personalized action steps to improve fitness levels. Some programs, such as Fitness for Life, use data to create personal action steps, but most teachers store away fitness testing scores and never look back. I have also found that many teachers only conduct fitness testing once each school year, so teachers and students are not provided with any feedback on their progress.

Does fitness testing in physical education motivate or encourage students to increase physical activity? Even if fitness scores are being used to create personal fitness plans, do the collected outcomes matter as much as the process or the steps required to live a healthy lifestyle? I would argue no. Most fitness testing standards compare students with their peers. Although there may be some validity to these standards, most kids who are in the lower percentiles already know that. These reminders may motivate some students to make positive changes, but for many others, placing a spotlight on their shortcomings in front of peers will drive them further away from adopting healthy habits. I believe helping students gain confidence in themselves while developing a positive relationship with physical activity by celebrating the process is much more effective in the long run.

Are fitness testing standards accurate indicators of wellness? Some objective-based fitness assessments are very reliable, while others can provide misleading results. If strength-based assessments do not include guidelines to ensure proper form is maintained, objective scores are meaningless. Who cares how many terrible push-ups a student can perform? Body mass index (BMI) is the most common method to collect body composition data in schools due to its convenience in comparison with reliable tests of body fat percentage, and it can also be a useful data point to monitor the overall wellness of large groups of people. Body mass index tends to serve as an accurate indicator of body composition in young children, in whom muscle mass is less prevalent; however, the imperfections of this measure among adolescents and adults have been widely discussed. For example, National Hockey League player Ryan McDonagh is listed as 6 ft, 1 in. (2 m) tall with a weight of 215 lb (98 kg) (figure 8.2). Although his teammates have been quoted as saying that "he doesn't have an ounce of fat on him" and his nickname is "Mack Truck" due to his muscular physique, his BMI is 28.4, which is on the high end of the overweight category (National Heart, Lung, and Blood Institute 2019). Although body composition is a critical

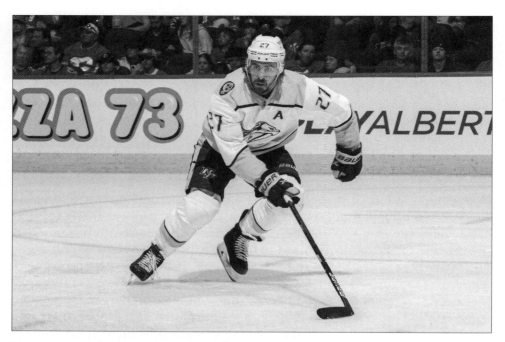

Figure 8.2 National Hockey League player Ryan McDonagh.
Gerry Thomas/NHLI via Getty Images

component of fitness and a key indicator of potential health risks, BMI is not always an accurate metric.

Considerations for Fitness Testing

Despite the fact that I do not recommend fitness testing in physical education, there are some important considerations for teachers who plan on implementing product-based fitness assessments. The FitnessGram by the Cooper Institute is a popular fitness testing program for physical education. Its slogan, "Learn, Assess, Address, Repeat," covers a lot of important bases that can potentially help students improve personal wellness. If PE teachers are going to conduct fitness testing, it is important that the following guidelines are prioritized.

- *Learn.* Incorporate instruction, skill development, and healthy lifestyle habits.
- *Assess.* Collect reliable, individualized data to determine personal needs, while considering student perception and peer interaction.
- *Address.* Create personalized fitness programs and process-based action steps to target individual needs.
- *Repeat.* Conduct further testing to determine the effectiveness of personalized plans, and provide additional feedback to modify future programming.

Assessment Types

A wide range of assessment options can be implemented in physical education to provide valuable feedback and measure performance. Assessments can be formal to calculate a grade or very informal to provide corrective feedback for students and allow teachers to check for understanding. Formative assessments are ongoing throughout a unit to provide feedback for future learning, while summative assessments take place at the end of a unit or marking period to provide a grade or progress report linked to overall achievement (figure 8.3).

Formative and summative assessments focusing on skill development and the process to achieve a healthy level of wellness should be embedded throughout fitness units. Three types of assessments that can be applied to fitness units are teacher, peer, and self-assessments.

Teacher Assessments

Teacher assessments are conducted by the teacher to provide feedback to students, check for understanding, and measure achievement for a grade. This type of assessment can be formative or summative to measure student achievement in three domains of learning: skill development (psychomotor), personal and social responsibility (affective), and cognitive learning. Quality checklists and rubrics will allow teachers to accurately assess student progress in all three domains.

Teacher Assessments in Action

Teacher assessments can take place at any point during a unit, including

- pre-assessments at the beginning of a unit to determine current ability level and retention from previous experiences,
- "ticket out the door" at the end of class to check for understanding,

Formative assessments:
Assessment for learning

When the chef tastes the soup

Summative assessments:
Assessment of learning

When the guests tastes the soup

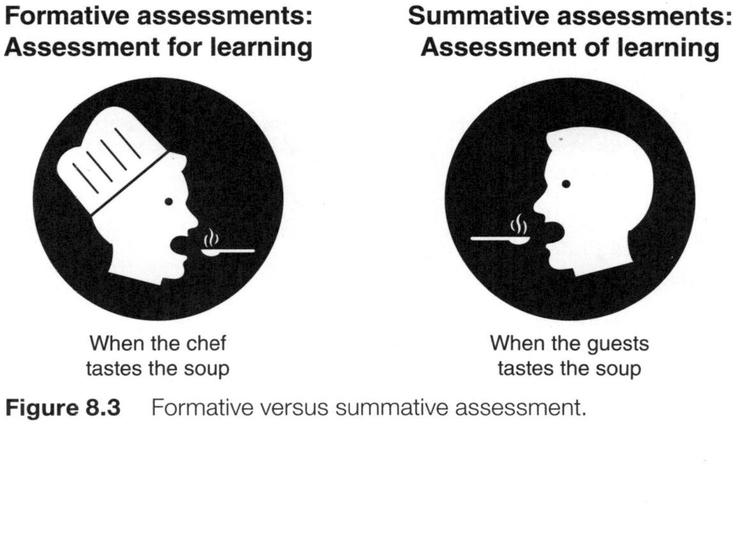

Figure 8.3 Formative versus summative assessment.

- formal summative assessments with checklists and rubrics for a grade or progress report,
- daily personal and social responsibility assessments, and
- written cognitive assessments.

Unfortunately, many teachers decide to forgo formal assessments because they are concerned that activity time will be sacrificed. In reality, formal assessments can take place at designated stations and during skill practice to maximize active participation.

Checklists and Rubrics

Checklists and rubrics do not need to be complicated. Basic checklists can simply consist of three to five skill cues previously introduced in class and a rubric to coordinate scoring. A sample functional strength training checklist with a rubric to conduct a formal assessment is shown in figure 8.4.

See the appendix and visit HK*Propel* for additional checklists that can be used for teacher-, peer-, and self-based skill assessments.

Teacher Assessment Record Keeping

Many methods to record and store assessment scores are available to teachers that will limit added administrative work, including the following:

- Entering scores directly into grading software using a portable device
- Entering scores on Google Forms or tracking assessments on form response sheets

Rubric for Teacher Assessment

4: Student performs 5 of 5 skill cues correctly and consistently
3: Student performs 4 of 5 skill cues correctly and consistently
2: Student performs 3 of 5 skill cues correctly and consistently
1: Student performs 2 or fewer skill cues correctly and consistently
0: Student does not attempt the skill

Free squat	Yes	Not yet
Heels are glued to the floor		
Sits back and taps the box		
Breaks the imaginary rubber band around the knees		
Shows off the logo on his or her shirt		
Smells the roses on the way down, blows out the candles on the way up		

Figure 8.4 Example rubric for functional strength training teacher assessment.

- Entering scores into Excel spreadsheets or Google Sheets
- Recording scores on printed team rosters
- Recording scores on individual student assessment cards

Peer Assessments

Formative peer assessments provide students with specific feedback from partners prior to summative teacher assessments, using practice checklists for guidance. Peer assessments are valuable to the partner receiving feedback because they enhance skill development. Additionally, students receive reinforcement of previously learned skills by evaluating others. Allowing students to analyze and evaluate peers meets a high level of learning, according to Bloom's Taxonomy (figure 8.5). Peer assessments also serve as a valuable behavior management tool by keeping students engaged between practice sets.

Peer Assessment in Action

Peer assessments can be implemented throughout a unit during skill practice sessions. I especially like using peer assessments during stations to provide additional feedback and to keep students engaged. Checklists can be posted at stations to help students provide specific verbal feedback to partners, or they can be printed for each group, allowing students to record practice assessment results. As shown in figure 8.6, the peer assessment checklist is the same as the teacher assessment checklist but without the rubric for scoring. Pictures with proper and improper form can also be used for younger populations.

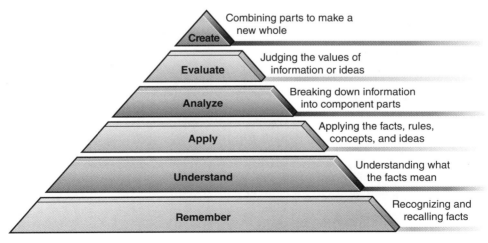

Figure 8.5 Bloom's taxonomy.

Checklist for Peer Assessment		
Free squat	Yes	Not yet
Heels are glued to the floor		
Sits back and taps the box		
Breaks the imaginary rubber band around the knees		
Shows off the logo on his or her shirt		
Smells the roses on the way down, blows out the candles on the way up		

Figure 8.6 Example peer-assessment checklist.

Using Peer Assessments to Provide Feedback
- If assessing students observe their partner performing a cue correctly, specific positive feedback can be provided.
- If assessing students observe a cue being performed incorrectly, they can provide specific corrective feedback.
- If a student is unable to perform a cue correctly after receiving specific corrective feedback, the assessing student will mark "not yet" on the checklist. Although this peer assessment has no impact on grading, the student performing the skill will know exactly what needs improvement for the future teacher assessment.

Self-Assessments

Self-analysis and evaluation are an extremely high level of learning. Although peer assessments can do wonders for skill development, having students watch themselves perform a skill while referring to a checklist or rubric takes motor learning to another level. Formative self-assessments can be implemented at any point throughout a unit to prepare students for summative teacher assessments.

Self-Assessment in Action

Teachers can easily plug self-assessments into stations or independent skill practice using the same checklists as peer assessments. The following are creative ways to have students analyze their own form:

- Students watch themselves in a mirror and refer to a checklist after each set.
- Students record a video on a personal device and refer to a checklist as they watch it back.
  - A partner can record the video, or students can use a tripod to record the video themselves.

- Teachers guide students through self-assessments using video analysis software on their device, such as *Coach's Eye* or many other user-friendly programs.
  - District policies should be reviewed before taking videos of students, either on personal or district-owned devices.

Personal and Social Responsibility

To assess student development in the affective domain, teachers must intentionally address a wide range of social-emotional learning (SEL) targets and create reliable rubrics and checklists to measure success. Teacher assessments and self-assessments can be implemented to evaluate personal and social responsibility on a daily basis and at specific benchmarks throughout a unit.

In addition to intentional SEL targets, many teachers conduct a daily personal and social responsibility assessment to reinforce general expectations and guidelines. Here is an example of a personal and social responsibility rubric for the fitness unit:

> *5 of 5: Students are prepared for class; participate in all activities, giving their best effort; demonstrate self-control and respect for others at all times; follow all safety rules while in the fitness center; and demonstrate appropriate fitness center etiquette.*

There are many amazing resources for creating personal and social responsibility assessments that meet the affective domain and SEL guidelines, including the Collaborative for Academic and Social Emotional Learning (CASEL) and QuaverEd.

Cognitive Assessment

Students require physical skills *and* knowledge to achieve and maintain a healthy lifestyle outside of school. If teachers focus solely on skill development and activity time during class, students will lack tools they need to be successful on their own. The following topics can be addressed with formative and summative assessments to determine if cognitive domain objectives are being met.

- Benefits of the activity
- Where to participate outside of school (community resources)
- Rules and etiquette
- Reinforcement of primary skills
- Situational concepts
- Authentic application of knowledge (program design)

Cognitive Assessments in Action

Cognitive assessments in physical education can include informal formative assessments to check for understanding and formal summative assessments to measure achievement at the end of a unit. Similar to the misconceptions surrounding formal skill assessments in physical education, many teachers are not willing to sacrifice activity time for cognitive assessments or are worried about adding the workload of grading and tracking scores. Teachers can check for understanding in a number of creative ways that limit time away from activities and lessen teacher workload, including the following:

- Think-pair-share partner discussions during class
- Ticket out the door
- Short Google Forms or Google Classroom
- Educational apps and online programs like Kahoot! and Plickers

Summative assessments to measure cognitive learning can consist of short hard-copy or online quizzes that do not require teachers to sacrifice a significant amount of activity or planning time. A quick 5- to 10-question quiz can be completed in just a few minutes during class, or independently. To limit additional administrative work, teachers can post quizzes in Google Classroom that are automatically graded and transferred to gradebooks in district-based programs like SchoolTool. This is a much better option than grading 100 to 200 paper quizzes during each unit, like in my early years in the field. Study guides can also be posted in Google Classrooms and other online programs to eliminate the need to print hard copies. Figure 8.7 provides an example of a short five-question quiz from a recent Victor Junior High School functional strength training unit. This quiz was completed on Google Classroom in 5 min at the beginning of class, then automatically graded and transferred to my grade book. The variety of teacher-friendly resources now available makes implementing cognitive assessments in physical education much easier than in the past.

Using Assessments to Calculate Physical Education Grades

Although some districts use assessments to create detailed progress reports that provide achievement-based feedback, many secondary schools have shifted to numeric grading in physical education. If students are receiving a numerical grade for physical education that is calculated with other subjects to determine an overall grade point average (GPA), it is imperative that teachers have reliable assessments and a valid record-keeping system in place to defend marking-period scores. Including grades in the overall

Functional Strength Training Quiz

1. Which statement does NOT describe functional strength training?
   a. strength training "with a purpose," related to daily activities and personal goals
   b. *isolating one muscle group at a time on a machine*
   c. using multiple muscle groups simultaneously
   d. using realistic movement patterns
2. Which of the following is a benefit of functional strength training?
   a. improves performance (strength, power, speed, balance, and coordination)
   b. decreases the risk of injury
   c. increases confidence and self-esteem
   d. *all of the above*
3. Which of the following is NOT a functional movement pattern?
   a. squat
   b. hip hinge
   c. *biceps curl*
   d. upper body pull
4. Which exercise is an example of a hip hinge movement pattern?
   a. push-up
   b. plank
   c. squat
   d. *kettlebell deadlift*
5. Where can you continue with functional strength training outside of PE?
   a. VCS after school, summer camps, JV or varsity athletics
   b. Next Level Strength and Conditioning
   c. Pinnacle
   d. *all of the above*

Figure 8.7 Sample Victor Junior High School functional strength training quiz.

GPA increases student accountability for learning and holds physical education on par with other subject areas.

Building-level departments have the ability to determine how assessments will be used to calculate marking-period grades. For students and parents to take skill development and cognitive learning in physical education seriously, most marking-period grades should be based on performance-centered achievement scores. This is how we break down marking-period grades for the functional strength training unit at Victor Junior High School:

- 60% physical performance
  - three grade-specific skill assessments (20% each)
- 20% cognitive learning
  - Unit quiz
- 20% personal and social responsibility
  - Average of daily personal and social responsibility assessments

There have been several occasions in my career when I have had to meet with the parents of less-skilled students to defend our grading structure because they were worried that their child's GPA would suffer due to the physical education grade. In my 20 years of teaching, I have never had a parent who was still hesitant about physical education being factored into the GPA after a quick explanation of why we emphasize performance, how assessments are geared toward the average student, and the level of support available for students who need extra help. In fact, most of these conversations end in parents praising our physical education program and our mission to guide students toward a healthy lifestyle.

What's Next

Part III of this book will go beyond teaching functional strength training in physical education to discuss how to apply functional strength training in other areas of your district, such as after-school programs and athletics. The next chapter will take a close look at facility design considerations to maximize the functional use of your space.

PART III

Functional Strength Training in Action

The third part of this book takes a deep dive into functional strength training beyond the classroom, because ultimately, what we want for students is to continue participating in functional strength training independently in order to achieve lifetime wellness and reach their personal goals. In chapters 9 through 11, I review a wide range of topics that will help PE teachers provide students with opportunities to apply what they learn in class on their own time, including facility design considerations, functional strength training program design guidelines, and advanced functional strength training for performance and athletics.

9

Facility Design

The differences between district fitness facilities can be as drastic as those between a sharp needle and a bowling ball. There are many factors that lead to this wide disparity between school facilities, including district priorities, the philosophy of those in charge, availability of space, and budgets. Many districts also fall victim to slick equipment salesmen who convince school officials that they need to fill their spaces with large, expensive selectorized machines. Some schools have multimillion-dollar fitness facilities that put many Division 1 colleges to shame, while others work out of closets or makeshift spaces with a hodgepodge of equipment. Regardless of the situation, every school has the ability to offer a quality functional strength training curriculum in physical education. Although each school will be faced with its own unique set of circumstances during the facility design and equipment selection process, there are several important guidelines that teachers and district officials must consider to optimize the space used for physical education and athletics.

Spatial Considerations

Over the years, I have visited countless schools to consult with district administrators during the facility design or update process. Just like when Brennan and Dale made bunk beds in the movie *Step Brothers*, my top priority is always open space—students need "room for activities." Although many athletic directors have a hard time parting ways with thousands of dollars' worth of selectorized machines, step one is always to clear out as many machines as possible and move all useful equipment to the walls. Open space in the middle of a facility offers a versatile teaching and training space that can be used for a wide range of activities.

Equipment Considerations

To stretch budgeted district funds as far as possible, it is important to prioritize equipment purchases that will allow teachers and coaches to offer quality programs without sacrificing valuable open space. Because district budgeting varies and space availability is not always consistent, I typically rank equipment purchases into three categories: equipment needs, equipment wants, and "utopia." Equipment priorities can change slightly over time based on many factors, but the following sections outline general itemized lists for each category based on my past experiences and current preferences.

Equipment Needs

Functional strength training skills can be taught in any open area with just a few free weights. Many skills can be introduced as body-weight movements, and external load can be added with a single kettlebell or dumbbell to increase intensity. Teachers can also use slow eccentric tempos and long isometric holds to increase intensity without a significant amount of external load. For teachers who have a limited budget, I would prioritize the following:

- Dumbbells (10-50 lb [5-23 kg]) or kettlebells (18-62 lb [8-28 kg])
- Purchasing pairs of dumbbells and ketttlebells is ideal if possible

The quantity of each item will depend on available funds. I suggest starting with middle-of-the-road weights and enough single free weights to break students into groups of two to four, based on class sizes.

Equipment Wants

Depending on budget, space availability, and class sizes, equipment wants may vary. I have listed items in preferential order for those who are unable to purchase all of them.

- Dumbbell pairs (5-85 lb [2-39 kg])
- Half racks with chin-up bars, weighted plates, and adjustable benches (two to five)
- Barbells and clips (two to five)
- Hex bars and clips (two to five)
- Soft-toss medicine balls (6-10 lb [3-5 kg])
- TRX or suspension trainers
- Agility ladders
- Foam plyometrics boxes
- PVC dowels for skill development (length: 5 ft [152 cm]; diameter: 1 in. [3 cm])

- Kettlebells (13-62 lb [6-28 kg]))
- Two to five sets of bumper plates (10-45 lb [5-20 kg])
- Covered resistance bands

Again, quantity will depend on budget, space, and class sizes. Consider how many of each item will be required to organize students in ideal groups of two to four. I suggest matching quantities of half racks, adjustable benches, barbells, and weighted plates to maximize use and facility flow.

"Utopia"

Utopia items are wish list items that would be great to add if money and space were of no concern, but they are not required to offer quality functional strength training programs in physical education. These items are in addition to the equipment wants previously listed.

- Dumbbell, barbell or hex bar, kettlebell, and medicine ball storage
- Foam rollers with storage
- Mini hurdles (6-12 in. [15-30 cm])
- Mini bands
- Training barbells (15 lb [17 kg])
- Dumbbell pairs (90-100 lb [41-45 kg]), double pairs (10-65 lb [5-30 kg])
- Half racks with chin-up bars, weighted plates, and adjustable benches (six or more)
- Barbells, clips (six or more)
- Hex bars, clips (six or more)
- Airex foam pads
- Rear foot elevated split squat (RFESS) stands
- Slideboards and boots
- Prowler sleds
- ANCORE cable systems
- Landmine sleeves
- Wind bikes
- Stability balls
- Ab wheels
- Six or more sets of bumper plates (10-45 lb [5-20 kg])
- Stackable blocks
- Safety squat bars
- Turf for mobility, sleds, and sprinting
- Just Jump mat
- Laser sprint timer

- Velocity-based training system
- Compact selectorized machines (one upper body push, one upper body pull, one leg press)
- General cardio equipment (treadmills, stationary bikes, stair steppers, elliptical machines)

Facility Flow

Even with an unlimited budget, open space must remain the priority. Quantity should be determined by how many pieces of each item are required to allow for ideal groups of two to four students, without sacrificing the open floor plan.

This section provides examples of high school fitness facilities that prioritize functional training equipment and open space (figures 9.1 and 9.2).

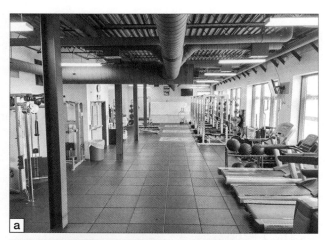

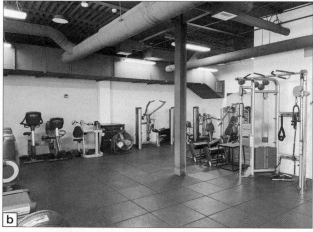

Figure 9.1 *(a)* Weight room and *(b)* cardio and selectorized machines at Victor High School (New York).

Perform Better! produces functional training and fitness equipment and offers facility design services. See figure 9.3 for a sample Perform Better! floor plan and pictures of the final product. Visit http://performbetter.com for more information.

To take a deeper dive into facility design, I recommend the book *Designing Strength Training Programs and Facilities* by Mike Boyle (2023).

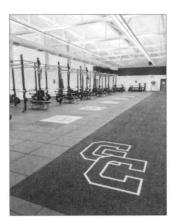

Figure 9.2 Gates Chili High School (New York).

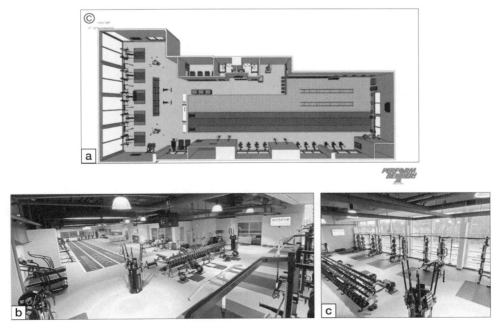

Figure 9.3 Perform Better! facility designs: *(a)* example from Boston Sports and *(b, c)* completed rooms.
Perform Better

What's Next

The next chapter will discuss program design for the general population. It will explore several factors that will allow students to design a functional strength training program to meet their specific goals and needs, including exercise selection, volume, intensity, how to organize a program, and more.

10

Program Design

Convincing students they should sacrifice their own time outside of school to participate in functional strength training programs and teaching them how to perform skills correctly is only the start of what should be prioritized in fitness units for secondary education. For students to achieve desired results independently, they must also possess the knowledge required to select exercises and organize workouts with appropriate volume and intensity.

It is important that teachers do not overload students with program design information. Remember that most students have limited experience with functional strength training. In most cases, complex sport performance programs will be far too advanced for students in the general population. Simple, full-body workouts performed with proper form and appropriate volume and intensity will yield significant results as students begin their fitness journeys with functional strength training. There are three major factors to consider when designing a functional strength training program: exercise selection, volume, and intensity.

Exercise Selection

Comprehensive full-body workouts are ideal for most students who will be strength training 2 to 3 days per week. Students can simply select one exercise appropriate for their ability level from each of the following movement-pattern or performance categories.

- Power
- Knee dominant
- Hip hinge
- Upper body push
- Upper body pull
- Core stability

It is ideal to perform exercises at submaximal power early in the workout when the nervous system is fresh. Exercises can be performed one at a time or paired together in complexes (two or more exercises performed in succession with limited rest). Using complexes can save time and keep students engaged during class. The sequence of exercises should be considered when working with advanced populations, but it is less critical for beginners.

Volume

The primary benefits of functional strength training for younger students are coordination and skill development. Improvements in strength, power, speed, and body composition are welcomed residual byproducts of quality training at this age. Specific repetition schemes that traditionally result in targeted physiological adaptations with older populations are less crucial with adolescents. Selecting sets and repetitions that will allow students to accumulate quality repetitions will stimulate the nervous system and reinforce motor learning. With middle-level and early high school students, I suggest prescribing 3 to 5 sets of 5 to 10 repetitions for each exercise to achieve the desired results.

Intensity

Basic progressive overload is all that students with limited strength training experience need in order to notice significant benefits. To simplify this concept, I tell students that the last repetition of each set should be perfect but challenging. If they are unable to perform the last repetition with proper form, the weight is obviously too heavy. If they feel that they could have done 5 more perfect repetitions at the selected weight, it isn't heavy enough. I suggest keeping exercises the same for at least 3 weeks before changing skill progressions if students are consistently following a structured program. When students notice greater ease, they can simply add 5 to 10 lb. This oversimplified progressive overload approach will lead to significant increases in strength, motor learning, and other facets of performance over time.

Individualized Modifications Based on Personal Goals and Ability Level

Teachers can provide younger students with programs and program templates, but personalized program design should be a major focal point for high school students approaching graduation to prepare them for a lifetime of success.

Middle School Program Design

The middle school program is very general, with no focus on individualized needs, because the primary goals for this age group are skill development and coordination, which are achieved by performing skills with proper form. Table 10.1 provides a simple template that middle school students can use to create their own functional strength training workouts by selecting their favorite skills from each category. Table 10.2 offers a bank of exercises for each category shown in table 10.1. These templates are available in HK*Propel*.

Table 10.1 **Sample Middle School Functional Strength Training Workout Template**

DAY 1	
Exercise	Sets × repetitions
A1) Power	3 × 5
A2) Knee dominant	3 × 5
A3) Upper body pull	3 × 10
Exercise	**Sets × repetitions**
B1) Hip hinge	3 × 5
B2) Upper body push	3 × 5
B3) Core stability	3 × 20 sec or 3 × 10 sec

From N. VanKouwenberg, *Functional Strength Training for Physical Education*. (Champaign, IL: Human Kinetics, 2025).

Table 10.2 **Exercise Bank**

Power	Knee dominant	Hip hinge	Upper body pull	Upper body push	Core
Split jump	Goblet squat	Hex deadlift	Chin-up *Assisted	BB bench	Side plank
MB throw	Free squat	KB deadlift	TRX row	Half-kneeling press	Bird dog
Box jump	Step-up	PVC RDL	BB inverted row	Push-up *Elevated	Plank

Abbreviations: BB = barbell; KB = kettlebell; MB = medicine ball; RDL = Romanian deadlift.
*Modified variation to perform with proper technique if needed.
From N. VanKouwenberg, *Functional Strength Training for Physical Education*. (Champaign, IL: Human Kinetics, 2025).

High School Program Design

Consistent with middle school program guidelines, high school students should create comprehensive full-body workouts that include at least one exercise from each movement pattern or performance category. High school students should have more exercises in their Rolodex to choose from due to previous experiences in physical education, but it is critical that selected variations are appropriate for each individual based on ability level. If a student is unable to perform a skill correctly because of functional limitations or other restrictions, exercises must be modified, or an alternate variation can be selected.

If students participate in functional strength training workouts consistently 2 to 3 days per week, they can either keep exercises the same each day or design two to three unique workouts to perform over the course of the week. Again, to maximize adaptation, I strongly recommend waiting at least 3 weeks before changing exercises.

Volume and intensity can be altered with advanced high school students to target individualized goals. Different repetition schemes and associated intensities can result in unique physiological adaptations. Students can either target specific results that are in line with their personal goals or cycle through different repetition schemes every 3 to 4 weeks to experience a wide range of benefits.

Here is a breakdown of program design considerations that can be presented to high school students in physical education.

- Select at least one exercise from each movement pattern or category for each workout
    - Power
    - Knee dominant
    - Hip hinge
    - Upper body push
    - Upper body pull
    - Core stability
- Begin with basic exercises and progress to more complex variations of each movement pattern or performance category every 3 to 4 weeks
- Select the desired training focus and prescribe appropriate volume and intensity (figure 10.1) (Schoenfeld et al. 2021)
    - Strength: 1 to 5 repetitions per set
    - Hypertrophy: 8 to 12 repetitions per set
    - Endurance: 15 or more repetitions per set

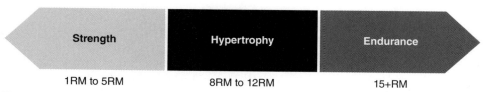

Figure 10.1 Strength training volume continuum.

- Perform 3 to 5 sets of 3 to 15 repetitions based on the desired outcome
- Power exercises should be performed at the beginning of each workout in sets of 3 to 5 repetitions, regardless of the training focus
- As repetitions (volume) decrease, weight (intensity) will increase and vice versa
- Gradually increase intensity as the current weight starts to feel easy, always prioritizing proper form
- Linear periodization: For comprehensive results over an extended period, cycle through training objectives in this order, switching every 3 to 4 weeks:
  - Hypertrophy
  - Strength
  - Maximum strength and power
- Complexes (optional) are short, 2- to 4-exercise circuits that will save time and maximize the productivity of a workout:
  - A1) Box jump 5 reps
  - A2) Front squat 5 reps
  - A3) Plank for 20 sec
  - Rest for 2 minutes; repeat 3 times

Visit HK*Propel* for example program designs and a downloadable program design template for secondary-level students.

What's Next

Although the primary focus of this book is to provide teachers with the tools they need to implement functional strength training in physical education, these concepts can also be applied to interscholastic athletics and sport performance programs. Many physical education teachers also coach sports and may be in charge of designing sport performance programs for their teams. The next chapter will focus on the unique factors that must be considered when designing functional strength training programs for athletes.

11

Connecting Functional Strength Training in Physical Education to Athletics

Implementing a sequential functional strength training curriculum in physical education can have a drastic impact on the quality of a district's sport-performance training programs. Athletes will require less instruction during training sessions because they will already possess a solid foundation of skills, knowledge, and general athleticism from previous experiences in physical education. This will allow district strength and conditioning coaches to focus more on leading productive, individualized training sessions without having to waste a significant amount of time on teaching exercises from scratch.

Goals of a Quality High School Strength and Conditioning Program

The goals of a high school strength and conditioning program should be to develop top-notch people, teammates, and athletes. There are many factors beyond the exercises, sets, and repetitions that separate the best high school programs from others. *Culture* can seem like an overplayed term at times, but there is nothing more important to the success of a high school strength and conditioning program. Elite high school strength and conditioning programs breed a culture that thrives on core values such as passion, school pride, dedication, and accountability. Athletes flock to the infectious environment that these powerful characteristics create.

Consistency is the big secret behind building elite high school athletes. The results that athletes can experience in high school are off the charts due to significant developmental advantages, and these results have more to do with showing up than with the X's and O's of training. Although comprehensive, science-driven sport performance training programs are important to maximize results and safety, getting athletes in the door consistently is the real secret sauce.

The following are specific goals of a quality high school strength and conditioning program:

- Developing character and leadership skills
- Promoting the value of consistent training
- Teaching good weight-room habits
- Further developing functional strength training and sport performance skills
- Offering quality training programs led by trained professionals
- Decreasing the risk of sport-related injury
- Improving all facets of sport performance by building well-rounded athletes

Extracurricular Sport Performance Program Design Guidelines

Consistent participation in a comprehensive functional strength training program with a focus on proper form and progressive overload will result in significant benefits that can be applied to any sport. However, additional training methods and considerations should be applied to sport performance programs to maximize results. To reach their full potential, athletes have more "buckets," or program focal points, to fill compared to the general population of PE students (figure 11.1). There are countless resources from the world's top strength and conditioning coaches that break down sport performance program design. The following basic compilation of guidelines is based on my personal experiences working with high school athletes.

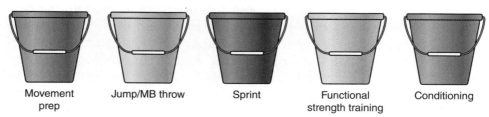

Figure 11.1 Sport performance buckets.

Sport Performance Program Considerations

Several factors that go beyond exercise selection, volume, and intensity must be considered when designing a sport performance program for athletes. When preparing a sport performance program, consider the following:

- Chronological age and training age of the population
- Training goals and sport-specific considerations
- In-season versus off-season training
- Functional needs or physical limitations of individual athletes
- Frequency and duration of training sessions
- Number of weeks with an athlete or team
- Equipment and space available
- Sport performance training skill level of athletes

Sport Performance Training Session Sequence

A sport performance training session should follow a specific sequence, including movement preparation, jumps and medicine ball (MB) throws, sprints, power, strength, and conditioning. This section provides considerations for each part of the sequence.

Movement Preparation

- Foam roller and soft-tissue quality
- Static stretching
- Joint-by-joint mobility
- Activation and prehab
- Dynamic stretching
- Low-level, explosive movements (ladder drills, basic jumps, hops, and leaps) and short, submaximal sprints to prime the nervous system

Jumps and MB Throws

- Implementation of meaningful jump, hop, leap, and plyometric progressions with appropriate volume (sets of 3 to 5 repetitions)
  - Progression from bilateral to unilateral variations
  - Progression of focus from landing and eccentric control to power output to rebounding
  - Filling of vertical, linear, lateral, and rotational exercise buckets each week when possible
- Implementation of a variety of MB throw variations over the course of a training program (sets of 3 to 5 repetitions)

Sprints

- Focus on maximum-effort sprinting with full recovery
- Gradual increase of sprint distances from 5 to 40 yd (5 to 37 m), with safe and intentional total sprint volumes
- Timing and recording of sprints, if possible, to increase intent, monitor readiness, and track progress over time
- Addition of meaningful sprint-start progressions, partner races, and short change-of-direction competitions in addition to timed sprints (or in place of them, if coaches do not have access to sprint timers)

Strength

- At least one exercise selected from each movement pattern or performance category
  - Power: aim for the middle third of the force-velocity curve with Olympic weightlifting variations, loaded jumps, and submaximal dynamic-strength exercises (sets of 3 to 5 repetitions)
  - Knee dominant: bilateral, unilateral, or frontal plane
  - Hip hinge: bilateral, unilateral, standing, or supine leg curl and hip lift
  - Upper body push: vertical, horizontal, or dynamic
  - Upper body pull: vertical, horizontal, or dynamic
  - Core stability: anti-extension, anti-rotation, anti–lateral flexion, or loaded carries
- Alternation of bilateral and unilateral or horizontal and vertical variations of the same movement pattern on opposite days, such as the following examples:
  - Day 1: bilateral front squat; day 2: split squat
  - Day 1: single-leg Romanian deadlift; day 2: hex deadlift
  - Day 1: barbell (BB) bench press; day 2: half-kneeling press
  - Day 1: one-arm row; day 2: chin-up
  - Day 1: plank; day 2: suitcase carry
- Selection of baseline variations in the group setting that are appropriate for roughly 80% of the group, regression of skills for individuals if needed, and use of progression lists to add complexity from phase to phase
- Pairing of two to four exercises in complexes that will keep athletes productive between sets of primary compound exercises

- Avoidance of system overload due to pairing grip-dominant exercises and heavy movements from the same pattern in one complex
- With advanced populations, incorporation of contrast training (post-activation potentiation) in the first strength complex to maximize muscle recruitment and power development by pairing a maximum-effort strength exercise with a submaximal power exercise in the same movement pattern
  - Example: BB bench press (4 sets of 3 repetitions [4 × 3]) paired with tall kneeling MB chest pass (4 × 3)
  - Example: farmer split squat (4 × 3) paired with continuous split jump (4 × 3)

Conditioning

This should be the first bucket to get cut if time is limited, due to sport-specific conditioning in practice and the ability for athletes to condition on their own. When focusing on conditioning, prioritize safety by considering overuse and the potential for form breakdown. Target specific energy systems with intentional work-to-rest ratios and gradually increase volume (Baechle and Earle 2008).

- Phosphagen (i.e., adenosine triphosphate and phosphocreatine system) (5 to 10 sec)
  - Work-to-rest ratio of 1:12 to 1:20
  - Wind-bike sprints, hill sprints, or sled sprints
- Fast glycolysis (15 to 30 sec)
  - Work-to-rest ratio of 1:3 to 1:5
  - Wind-bike sprints, shuttles, heavy sled march or drag, or MB slams
- Fast glycolysis and oxidation (1 to 3 min)
  - Work-to-rest ratio of 1:3 to 1:4
  - Submaximal bike sprints, submaximal tempo runs, submaximal circuits, or submaximal slideboard
- Oxidative (>3 min)
  - Work-to-rest ratio of 1:1 to 1:3
  - Constant-state bike, run, or swim

See table 11.1 for three different performance buckets that can be filled over the course of a comprehensive sport performance program for each movement pattern and performance focus.

Table 11.1 **Examples of Different Movement Pattern or Performance Category "Buckets"**

Pattern or focus	Bucket 1	Bucket 2	Bucket 3
Jump, hop, or leap	Vertical	Lateral or rotational	Unilateral
Medicine ball	Chest pass	Shot put or punch	Rotational or scoop
Power	Olympic variations	Bilateral loaded jumps with reset	Continuous bilateral loaded jumps
Knee dominant	Bilateral	Unilateral	Frontal plane
Hip hinge	Bilateral	Unilateral	Supine hip lift or leg curl
Upper body push	Vertical	Horizontal	Power or dynamic
Upper body pull	Vertical	Horizontal	Power or dynamic
Core stability	Anti-extension	Anti-rotation or anti-lateral flexion	Loaded carry
Conditioning	Phosphagen	Glycolysis	Oxidative

Volume and Intensity Selection

Many coaches overthink volume and intensity with high school athletes. If athletes perform 3 to 5 sets of 5 to 10 repetitions (total of 15 to 30 repetitions per strength exercise or workout), gradually increasing resistance over time, they will experience significant results. In order to maximize power output and maintain proper form, power exercises should not exceed sets of 3 to 5 repetitions.

Linear periodization is one basic approach coaches can use during the off-season if they will be working with athletes for more than 8 weeks. There are a variety of approaches to implementing linear periodization with off-season high school athletes. In some cases, volume can remain fairly constant over the course of a 3- to 4-week phase as intensity gradually increases, or intensity can remain fairly constant as volume gradually increases. Regardless, the goal is to perform skills with perfect form and gradually increase the demand over the course of the training program.

The following is one approach to linear periodization that I have found to be successful when working with high school athletes over an extended period of time.

- Phase 1: hypertrophy
  - 2 to 3 sets of 8 to 12 repetitions, for 20 to 30 total repetitions per strength exercise (examples: 2 × 10, 2 × 12, 3 × 8, or 3 × 10 repetitions)
- Phase 2: strength
  - 3 to 4 sets of 5 to 6 repetitions, for 15 to 20 total repetitions per strength exercise (examples: 3 × 5, 3 × 6, or 4 × 5 repetitions)
- Phase 3: maximum strength and power
  - 3 to 5 sets of 3 to 4 repetitions, for 9 to 16 total repetitions per exercise (examples: 3 × 3, 3 × 4, 4 × 3, 4 × 4, or 5 × 3 repetitions)

The number of repetitions should stay the same for the first 3 weeks of a phase, gradually increasing weight as the final repetitions of each set become easier (progressive overload). Decrease repetitions to deload during week 4 before progressing exercise variations and changing repetition schemes. Intensity will increase as volume decreases, and intensity will decrease as volume increases. Slow-eccentric-tempo exercises and isometric holds (5 sec × 3 repetitions) can be added to one or two primary exercises per day during the hypertrophy phase. Add eccentric-tempo exercises to the first 2 weeks of the phase, followed by isometric holds during weeks 3 and 4. Rate-of-perceived-exertion scales, one-repetition-maximum percentages, and/or velocity-based training can be used to increase intent and meaningful intensity selection.

In-Season Considerations

The goal of an in-season sport performance program is to help athletes enter the postseason in peak performance and health. Many sport coaches and athletes dismiss the importance of in-season training and either skip it altogether or go through the motions to check a box. Despite the busy schedules and physical demands that come along with a high school sport season, as little as 30 min per week of quality in-season training can pay massive dividends down the stretch. It amazes me that some coaches and athletes will sacrifice endless hours on practice, film, scouting, and off-season training but refuse to devote 30 min a week to something that could potentially make or break their season. Debunking common misconceptions and preaching the benefits of in-season training to coaches, athletes, and parents can go a long way in creating a culture that values year-round sport performance training.

For athletes to continue to make gains in strength, power, and speed over the course of a long season while combating the risk of sport-related injury, the following factors must be considered when designing in-season programs.

- Overall workload, including practices, games, position-specific demands, and in-season workouts, to prevent overtraining
- Common sport-specific injuries
- In-season scheduling, including game days, practice times, and other time-consuming commitments
- Nutrition, hydration, sleep, lifestyle choices, stress management, and mental and emotional health

In-season sport performance programs must be very fluid and individualized to meet the specific needs of each team and athlete throughout the season. Strength and conditioning coaches must be prepared to make many last-minute modifications based on a combination of these factors. Making adjustments to intensity, volume, and exercise variations on the fly needs to be expected. Here are some general guidelines for designing a quality in-season sport performance program.

- Focus on what athletes are *not* doing in their sport.
  - In most cases, athletes are practicing or playing games 6 days a week. They are performing sport-specific movements hundreds if not thousands of times each day. Beating a dead horse by adding more of the same in the weight room can lead to overtraining and decreased performance when it counts. The main component of performance that most athletes do not address during practices and games is strength. A common misconception is that athletes will be sore for games if they strength train during the season. Some people also believe that in-season strength training should consist of high-volume, low-intensity workouts. In reality, by designing in-season programs that consist of primary compound exercises with low volume and moderate to high intensity, athletes will be filling a conditioning bucket that does not get addressed while playing their sport. The term *use it or lose it* applies perfectly to in-season strength maintenance and development. It is OK to lift heavy during the season if volume is low, proper form is maintained, and athletes are prioritizing recovery on their own time. Building strength during the season will not only decrease the risk of sport-related injury deep into the postseason but will also improve other facets of performance, such as power and speed, during game play. Two to four sets of 3 to 5 repetitions, with a total of 8 to 15 repetitions for each movement pattern, is recommended.
  - Unless teams have days off from practice during the week, there is no need to add conditioning to in-season training. The conditioning bucket is often already full to the brim from daily sport-specific demands.
- Target common sport-specific injuries by implementing combative prehab exercises within daily prepractice warm-ups, in-season training-movement preparation, and strength complexes.
- Monitor recovery and readiness by tracking weekly vertical jumps or using general wellness surveys to determine if it would be more beneficial to decrease the volume of strength training or substitute a recovery-focused workout on occasion. If athletes are not recovering well, be sure to have conversations about the importance of nutrition, hydration, sleep, lifestyle choices, stress management, mental and emotional health, and time management.

See the appendix of this book and visit *HKPropel* for sample off-season and in-season high school sport performance programs.

Additional Resources and Sport Performance Programming Systems

There is a wide variety of advanced programming methods and periodization systems that I would recommend for advanced athletes who have been training for 3 years or longer, including undulating block and conjugate periodization systems. Although there may be high school athletes who are high-profile Division 1 recruits, many of them are still newborns when it comes to training age. In most cases, even the most talented high school athletes will benefit a great deal from basic linear periodization with progressive overload. Here is a list of additional resources to take a deeper dive into sport-performance programming for beginner and advanced athletes.

- *New Functional Training for Sports* (Boyle 2016)
- *Designing Strength Training Programs and Facilities* (Boyle 2023)
- *Movement Over Maxes: Developing the Foundation for Baseball Performance* (Dechant 2018)
- *Triphasic Training: A Systematic Approach to Elite Speed and Explosive Strength Performance* (Dietz and Peterson 2012)
- *Physical Preparation for Ice Hockey* (Donskov, 2016)
- *The Gain, Go, Grow Manual: Programming for High Performance Hockey Players* (Donskov 2020)

Strength and Conditioning Certification Recommendations

If you are reading this book, you must have an interest in implementing functional strength training in PE fitness units or strength and conditioning programs in your district. Although a fitness or strength and conditioning certification is not required to achieve this goal, with the road map outlined in previous chapters, I strongly recommend that teachers who would like to take the lead on improving districtwide programs continue to grow as professionals in this area. The more ammunition you have to make educated decisions, have discussions with other teachers, and influence policy change with district administrators, the better. If you are interested in becoming a certified strength and conditioning coach or fitness professional, several certifications are available. There are many factors to consider when deciding which certification to pursue. These are the top three options that I would recommend, with some general suggestions based on my personal experiences.

Certified Functional Strength Coach (CFSC). I received my CFSC certification several years ago. I decided to go in this direction because it is more than just letters after my name. Mike Boyle and his team created this certification to fill the gap between fitness knowledge and the ability to effectively communicate as a strength and conditioning coach. The course consists of valuable information that is applicable to coaching fitness classes and strength and conditioning sessions and that I still use every day. The coursework covers a wide range of topics, including exercise science, functional anatomy, communication skills, program design, and skill development, to ensure that coaches are able to properly demonstrate exercises and offer individualized modifications when necessary. The final assessment includes an online exam and a practical coaching component that requires participants to demonstrate skills correctly and modify variations on the spot. I have recommended the CFSC certification to several PE teachers and young strength and conditioning coaches over the years. Regardless of their previous experience in the field, they were provided with adequate resources and hands-on skill development training to pass the certification, and more importantly, they walked away with the tools they needed to successfully help others. Visit http://certifiedfsc.com to learn more.

Certified Strength & Conditioning Specialist (CSCS). The CSCS has been the gold standard of strength and conditioning certifications for many years. This accredited certification from the National Strength and Conditioning Association (NSCA) is recognized as the preferred certification for major organizations like the National Collegiate Athletics Association. Certification requirements include prerequisite college degrees, passing a written examination consisting of scientific foundations and practical and applied competencies, and ongoing continuing education credits. Visit the certification section at http://nsca.com to learn more.

USA Weightlifting (USAW). The USAW certifications apply Olympic weightlifting skills and concepts to sport performance training, general fitness, and competitive Olympic weightlifting. This certification requires the completion of a 2-day course that covers science-based concepts, skill development, effective coaching techniques, assessment, program design, and more. Visit the weightlifting section at www.teamusa.org to learn more.

Closing Remarks

Thank you for taking the time to read *Functional Strength Training for Physical Education*. Refer to the appendix of this book and online material in HK*Propel* for a wide range of valuable materials that can be used to transform your fitness units and high school strength and conditioning programs.

As physical educators, we have the ability to influence students beyond our time with them. It is our responsibility to help students by providing the tools they need to maintain a healthy lifestyle into adulthood, even if it requires extra time and work. I am hopeful that with this easy-to-follow road map, teachers will expose students to the lifelong benefits of functional strength training in physical education!

Appendix: Functional Strength Training for PE Resources

This portion of the book includes example resources for PE teachers to successfully design and implement quality functional strength training units and extracurricular activities, regardless of previous experience and knowledge in this area. The resources provided here include external skill cues, a sample curriculum map, a personalized curriculum design template, assessment checklists, sample functional strength training, and sport performance programs.

These resources are also provided in HK*Propel* as downloadable forms that you may print and use in your own practice.

Sample K-12 Curriculum Map and Design Template

There are endless examples of quality K-12 functional strength training curriculum maps. As long as teachers follow developmentally appropriate skill progressions, there is no right or wrong approach. Table A.1 shows an example of a K-12 functional strength training curriculum map that would be ideal for teachers who have blended grades or would like to dedicate more than 1 year to working on primary skills.

Table A.1 **Sample K-12 Curriculum Map**

Grade	Knee dominant	Hinge	Upper body push	Upper body pull	Power	Core	Concepts
11-12	Split squat or RFESS	Skater Squat	DB bench press (incline or flat)	Chin-up or pull-up	Hang power clean	Stability ball rollout	Resources, program design
9-10	Front squat	Single-leg RDL	BB bench press	Standing 1-arm DB row	Hang clean pull or hang high pull	Staggered side plank	FITT principles: volume and intensity
7-8	Goblet squat	KB or hex bar deadlift	Half-kneeling DB or KB press	Tall kneeling pull-down	Broad jump	Bird dog	Why FST, exercise selection
5-6	Free squat	Hip hinge or PVC RDL	Push-up	Inverted or TRX row	Box jump	Plank	5 Components of fitness and why FST

From N. VanKouwenberg, *Functional Strength Training for Physical Education*. (Champaign, IL: Human Kinetics, 2025).

Elementary	Speed and agility	Flexibility	Coordination	Strength
3-5	Tag games Relay races Obstacle courses Short sprints	Introduce basic stretching, mobility, and gymnastics	Introduce ladder drills, jump rope, and contralateral coordination exercises including • Deadbugs • Opposition bear crawls • Additional skipping variations	Introduce external skill cues to basic functional exercises in warm-ups and stations, including • Toe touch to squat • Snap-down or hinge • Plank • Elevated push-ups • Step-up • Inverted row
K-2	Tag games Relay races Obstacle courses	Expose students to a wide range of movements at different levels (over and under objects) and in a variety of planes of motion during obstacle courses and other games	Introduce gross motor skills including marching, galloping, skipping, lateral shuffling, and hopping	Incorporate elementary-level functional strength progressions within obstacle courses and other games

Abbreviations: BB = barbell; DB = dumbbell; FITT = frequency, intensity, type, and time; FST = functional strength training; KB = kettlebell; RDL = Romanian deadlift; RFESS = rear foot elevated split squat.

From N. VanKouwenberg, *Functional Strength Training for Physical Education*. (Champaign, IL: Human Kinetics, 2025).

Use the blank template provided in HK*Propel* to design your own K-12 functional strength training curriculum map.

External Skill Cues for Primary Functional Skill Progressions

In tables A.2 to A.7, I have listed some of my favorite external skill cues for the primary exercises in the K-12 curriculum map example, along with commonly used modifications and variations.

Table A.2 **Knee Dominant Exercise External Skill Cues**

Free squat	Goblet squat	Front squat	Split squat or RFESS
Heels are glued to the floor	Hold the dumbbell vertically with your palms up; attach it to your shirt collar	Release your thumb and pinky finger to create a shelf with your arms for the bar to sit on	Split your feet in front of and behind a small pad, with your back heel up like you have a tack in it
Sit back and tap the box, so your body looks like a lightning bolt from the side (lower leg, upper leg, torso)*	Protect your ribs with your elbows, like a boxer	Point flashlights on your elbows to the front wall	Lower your back knee to the pad and tap it without breaking the bubble wrap
Break the imaginary band on your knees	Heels are glued to the floor	Squeeze a large grapefruit between your elbows	Drive your front foot through the floor back to the starting position
Show off the logo on your shirt	Sit back and tap the box, with your elbows inside your knees	Sit back and tap the box, with your heels glued to the floor	RFESS: Place your laces on an RFE rack or bench

Abbreviations: RFE = rear foot elevated; RFESS = rear foot elevated split squat.

*To assist if unable to squat to a small box with proper form, place a small board or plate under the heels.

From N. VanKouwenberg, *Functional Strength Training for Physical Education*. (Champaign, IL: Human Kinetics, 2025).

Table A.3 **Hip Hinge Exercise External Skill Cues**

PVC RDL or hinge	KB or hex deadlift	SL RDL	Skater squat
Hold the PVC, dowel, or BB with your hands outside of your legs and push your knuckles to the floor	Chop your hips back; reach with straight arms to make a YouTube play button (triangle) in the middle of your body	Stand on one foot with a soft knee; balance like you're on a boat in rough water	Stand on one foot with one or two pads stacked behind your opposite leg
With soft knees, pull the bar into your legs like you're trying to make a mark	Make a double chin and keep a neck brace on throughout each repetition	Reach your opposite heel to the back wall and reach your opposite hand to the front wall, or the hold DB or KB straight down to the floor	Squeeze a tennis ball (imaginary or real) in the back of the opposite knee
Scrape the bar down your legs until it's below your knees; try to touch your tailbone to the back wall	Brace yourself like someone is going to tackle you	Turn your back pinky toe in toward the floor to keep your hips level	Lower your opposite knee to the pad without touching the floor with your foot; press light weight out as you lower your knee
Stand up tall like you're getting measured	Push your feet through the floor and stand up tall like you're getting measured*	Stand up tall like you're getting measured	Gently tap the pad without breaking the bubble wrap; stand up tall to the starting position

Abbreviations: DB = dumbbell; KB = kettlebell; RDL = Romanian deadlift; RFESS = rear foot elevated split squat; SL = single leg.

*To assist if unable to keep the back flat, elevate the KB or hex bar off the ground.

From N. VanKouwenberg, *Functional Strength Training for Physical Education*. (Champaign, IL: Human Kinetics, 2025).

Table A.4 **Upper Body Push Exercise External Skill Cues**

Push-up	Half-kneeling press	BB bench press	DB bench press
Place your hands under your shoulders with your belly button up, and tuck your tail like a board is on your back*	Place one knee on a pad with the opposite knee up, balancing a glass of water on your front leg	Lie on the bench with your forehead under the bar and the spotter behind you	Lie on the bench with your palms facing each other and the top of the DB at your armpits
Lower your chest and tap a small pad on the floor (real or imaginary)	Drive your flat front foot into the ground and tuck in your back toe	Lock out your elbows over your chest, trying to bend the bar	Push the DB through the ceiling while rotating the tops of the dumbbells toward each other and your palms away from you
From above, your arms should look like an arrow, or an "A" for awesome (not a "T" for terrible)	On the knee-down side, your hand holds the DB or KB with your palm to your ear, like you're on the phone	Pull the bar down until it lightly taps the logo on your shirt	Pull the DB back to the starting position with your palms facing each other
Push the floor away from you to return to the starting position	Punch the DB or KB through the ceiling while squeezing a tennis ball in your opposite hand (real or imaginary)	Push the bar through the ceiling until your elbows are locked	Incline DB bench: use the same cues, but incline the adjustable bench 30-40 degrees

Abbreviations: BB = barbell; DB = dumbbell; KB = kettlebell.

To assist, elevate the hands to a bench, box, or barbell in rack.

From N. VanKouwenberg, *Functional Strength Training for Physical Education*. (Champaign, IL: Human Kinetics, 2025).

Table A.5 Upper Body Pull Exercise External Skill Cues

TRX or inverted row	Tall kneeling pull-down	Standing 1-arm row	Chin-up variations
Dig your heels into the ground, point your toes to the ceiling, and attach a board to your back	Stand tall on your knees, with your hips and knees under your shoulders	Stand an arm's length away from a bench with your feet wide, like you're riding a horse	Grab the bar or rack with your palms facing you and your knuckles out (chin-up), with your palms facing each other (neutral chin-up), or with your palms out and your knuckles facing you (pull-up)
Start with your arms locked and your thumbs down	Reach up and grab the band or rope cable attachment with your thumbs facing each other	Chop your hips back, push one hand into the bench like a football stiff arm, and pick up a DB or KB with the other hand	Start with your arms locked like you're hanging off a cliff
Pull the logo on your shirt to your hands and rotate your thumbs to your armpits	Pull the band or rope cable attachment to the logo on your shirt, with your thumbs pointing to your armpits	Level your hips and flatten your back like you have a glass of water on it	Pull the collar of your shirt to the bar or rack while the rest of your body stays frozen
Inverted row: Line up the logo on your shirt under the bar with your knuckles up; pull the logo on your shirt to the bar Assisted: The taller you stand, or the farther your hands are from the ground, the easier it will be	Squeeze a $100 bill in your armpits before slowly returning to the starting position	Pull your wrist to your ribs without letting the glass of water fall off, then slowly lower to the starting position	Assisted: Attach a superband to the bench press clips on the rack to stand on, or loop around the chin-up bar to place around your foot

Abbreviations: DB = dumbbell; KB = kettlebell.

From N. VanKouwenberg, *Functional Strength Training for Physical Education*. (Champaign, IL: Human Kinetics, 2025).

Table A.6 Power Exercise External Skill Cues

Box jump	Broad jump	Hang clean or high pull	Hang power clean
Swing your arms back and drop your hips to prepare for takeoff	Swing your arms and push your hips back to prepare for takeoff	Stand with soft knees, holding the BB outside of your legs; curl your knuckles under the bar like a gorilla	Stand with soft knees, holding the BB outside of your legs; curl your knuckles under the bar like a gorilla
Swing your arms up and try to jump through the ceiling	Swing your arms forward and try to jump through the front wall	Pull the bar into your leg and scrape your thigh until you hit the top of your knee	Pull the bar into your leg and scrape your thigh until you hit the top of your knee
Land on the box softly, slowly, and quietly, like a helicopter, or like you're landing on bubble wrap or thin ice	Land softly, slowly, and quietly like a ninja, or how a car comes to a stop sign	Drive the top of your head through the ceiling like you're jumping, but your toes are stuck to the floor	Drive the top of your head through the ceiling like you're jumping; pull the bar to your shirt collar with your knuckles facing the ground
Your body should look the same during the landing and takeoff, or the box height should be adjusted	Jump from and land on both feet equally	Hang clean pull: Keep your arms locked Hang high pull: Pull the bar to your shirt collar with your knuckles facing the ground	Quickly drop under the bar with your hips back, and imagine flashlights on your elbows pointing at the front wall to create a shelf for the bar to sit on

Abbreviation: BB = barbell.

From N. VanKouwenberg, *Functional Strength Training for Physical Education*. (Champaign, IL: Human Kinetics, 2025).

Table A.7 **Core Exercise External Skill Cues**

Plank	Bird dog	Staggered side plank	Stability ball rollout
Balance on your elbows and toes with your belly button toward the ceiling and your tail tucked	Make a flat tabletop with your back while on your hands and knees	Anchor one elbow to the ground, facing sideways; split your feet like scissors, with the top leg forward	Stand tall on your knees with your arms locked and your hands together like you're going to cut the ball in half
Make a double chin so your body looks like a board or plank from head to feet	Reach out with your opposite arm and leg, like you're taking two legs of the table away	Pick your hips up, push them in, and make a double chin so your body is as straight as a board from head to feet	Slowly fall forward, rolling the ball up the bottoms of your arms
Place your hands flat on the floor (stay on your elbows) and pull the floor to your feet	Keep your back flat and your hips level, like you have a glass of water on your back	Raise your top arm to the sky, squeeze a tennis ball (real or imaginary) in your top hand, and brace like you're in a hurricane	Keep your tail tucked and your back flat like a board
Brace yourself like you're in a hurricane	Return all four legs of the table to the ground and repeat on the opposite side	Switch sides	Pull your body back to the tall kneeling starting position while keeping your back flat like a board

From N. VanKouwenberg, *Functional Strength Training for Physical Education*. (Champaign, IL: Human Kinetics, 2025).

Teacher, Peer, and Self-Assessment Checklists

As discussed in chapter 8, checklists can simply consist of three to five designated skill cues focusing on the process, or proper technique, of an exercise. These checklists can be used to conduct teacher and peer assessments and student self-assessments. Associated rubrics can be created to provide a numerical score for progress reports or unit grades. In this section, I have included examples of four cue checklists for each skill listed in the K-12 curriculum map, which can be used with the following four-point rubric to conduct teacher assessments for progress reports and to calculate numerical grades.

4: Student performs 4 of 4 skill cues correctly and consistently
3: Student performs 3 of 4 skill cues correctly and consistently
2: Student performs 2 of 4 skill cues correctly and consistently
1: Student performs 1 of 4 skill cues correctly and consistently
0: Student does not attempt the skill

Knee Dominant Exercise Checklists

Knee dominant: Free squat	Yes	Not yet
Heels are glued to the floor		
Sits back and taps the box		
Breaks the imaginary band around the knees		
Shows off the logo on his or her shirt		

From N. VanKouwenberg, *Functional Strength Training for Physical Education*. (Champaign, IL: Human Kinetics, 2025).

Knee dominant: Goblet squat	Yes	Not yet
Dumbbell is vertical and connected to the shirt collar, and the palms are up		
Elbows protect ribs like a boxer		
Heels are glued to the floor		
Sits back and taps the box with elbows inside knees		

From N. VanKouwenberg, *Functional Strength Training for Physical Education*. (Champaign, IL: Human Kinetics, 2025).

Knee dominant: Front squat	Yes	Not yet
Elbows point forward to create a shelf for the bar		
Elbows are in, like squeezing a large grapefruit		
Heels are glued to the floor		
Sits back and taps the box, breaking the imaginary band on the knees		

From N. VanKouwenberg, *Functional Strength Training for Physical Education*. (Champaign, IL: Human Kinetics, 2025).

Knee dominant: Split squat	Yes	Not yet
One foot is in front of the pad and one is behind		
Back heel is up		
Slowly lowers the back knee to the pad and taps lightly		
Drives the front foot through the floor to the starting position		

From N. VanKouwenberg, *Functional Strength Training for Physical Education*. (Champaign, IL: Human Kinetics,

Hip Hinge Exercise Checklists

Hip hinge: PVC Romanian deadlift	Yes	Not yet
Hands are outside of the legs; arms are locked		
With soft knees, pulls the bar into the upper leg		
Pushes the hips back and scrapes the bar down the thigh until below the knee		
Stands up tall, as if getting measured		

From N. VanKouwenberg, *Functional Strength Training for Physical Education*. (Champaign, IL: Human Kinetics, 2025).

Hip hinge: Kettlebell or hex bar deadlift	Yes	Not yet
Chops the hips back; reaches down to make a triangle in the middle of the body		
Makes a double chin with a neck brace on		
Braces at the bottom, as if about to get tackled		
Pushes the feet through the floor, standing up tall as if getting measured		

From N. VanKouwenberg, *Functional Strength Training for Physical Education*. (Champaign, IL: Human Kinetics, 2025).

Hip hinge: Single-leg Romanian deadlift	Yes	Not yet
Balances on one foot with soft knees, as if on a boat		
Reaches the opposite heel to the back wall		
Turns the back pinky toe in to keep the hips level and the back flat		
Stands up tall, as if getting measured		

From N. VanKouwenberg, *Functional Strength Training for Physical Education*. (Champaign, IL: Human Kinetics, 2025).

Hip hinge: Skater squat	Yes	Not yet
Stands on one foot with one or two pads behind opposite knee		
Lowers the opposite knee; lightly taps the pad without touching the foot to the floor		
Presses light weight out while lowering the knee		
Stands up tall, as if getting measured		

From N. VanKouwenberg, *Functional Strength Training for Physical Education*. (Champaign, IL: Human Kinetics, 2025).

Upper Body Push Exercise Checklists

Upper body push: Push-up	Yes	Not yet
The hands are under the shoulders, the tail is tucked, and the back is flat like a board		
Lowers the chest and lightly taps the pad		
The arms look like an arrow or an "A" from above		
Pushes the floor (or elevated surface) away to the starting position with a flat back		

From N. VanKouwenberg, *Functional Strength Training for Physical Education*. (Champaign, IL: Human Kinetics, 2025).

Upper body push: Half-kneeling press	Yes	Not yet
One knee is down on the pad, the opposite knee is up, and the back toes are tucked		
The knee-side hand holds the dumbbell with the palm in, as if on the phone		
Presses the dumbbell as if punching it through the ceiling, until the arm is locked		
Makes a fist, as if squeezing a ball in the opposite hand		

From N. VanKouwenberg, *Functional Strength Training for Physical Education*. (Champaign, IL: Human Kinetics, 2025).

Upper body push: Barbell bench press	Yes	Not yet
Lies on the back with the forehead under the bar and the spotter behind the bench		
Locks elbows, with the bar over the logo on his or her shirt; tries to bend the bar		
Pulls the bar down and lightly taps the logo on his or her shirt		
Pushes the bar through the ceiling until the elbows are locked		

From N. VanKouwenberg, *Functional Strength Training for Physical Education*. (Champaign, IL: Human Kinetics, 2025).

Upper body push: Dumbbell bench press	Yes	Not yet
Lies on the back with the top of the dumbbell pointing toward the armpits		
Pushes the dumbbell through the ceiling until the arms are locked		
Rotates the tops of the dumbbells toward each other and the palms away at the top		
Pulls the dumbbell back to the starting position, with the top of the dumbbell pointing toward the armpit		

From N. VanKouwenberg, *Functional Strength Training for Physical Education*. (Champaign, IL: Human Kinetics, 2025).

Upper Body Pull Exercise Checklists

Upper body pull: TRX row	Yes	Not yet
Heels are down, toes are up, and the body is as straight as a board		
Arms start locked, with the thumbs down		
Pulls the logo on his or her shirt to the hands, rotating the thumbs to the armpits		
Lowers to the starting position, with the body as straight as a board		

From N. VanKouwenberg, *Functional Strength Training for Physical Education*. (Champaign, IL: Human Kinetics, 2025).

Upper body pull: Tall kneeling pull-down	Yes	Not yet
Stands tall on two knees, with the hips and knees under the shoulders		
Reaches up to grab the band or rope, with the thumbs facing each other		
Pulls the band or rope down, with the thumbs pointing at the armpits		
Squeezes a $100 bill in the armpits before returning to the starting position		

From N. VanKouwenberg, *Functional Strength Training for Physical Education*. (Champaign, IL: Human Kinetics, 2025).

Upper body pull: Standing 1-arm dumbbell row	Yes	Not yet
Starts an arm's length from the bench with the feet wide; chops the hips back		
Pushes one hand into the bench with a stiff arm and picks up the dumbbell with the other hand		
Pulls the wrist holding the dumbbell to the ribs		
The back stays flat, like balancing a glass of water		

From N. VanKouwenberg, *Functional Strength Training for Physical Education*. (Champaign, IL: Human Kinetics, 2025).

Upper body pull: Chin-up (neutral chin-up, pull-up)	Yes	Not yet
Grabs the bar or rack palms in (chin-up), facing each other (neutral chin-up), or facing out (pull-up)		
Starts with straight arms, like hanging from a cliff		
Pulls the collar of his or her shirt to the bar or rack, with the rest of the body frozen		
Uses an appropriate level of assistance to maintain proper form, if needed		

From N. VanKouwenberg, *Functional Strength Training for Physical Education*. (Champaign, IL: Human Kinetics, 2025).

Power Exercise Checklists

Power: Box jump	Yes	Not yet
Swings the arms back and drops the hips before takeoff		
Swings the arms up, attempting to jump through the ceiling		
Lands slowly, softly, and quietly on the box, like landing on bubble wrap		
The body position on landing matches takeoff		

From N. VanKouwenberg, *Functional Strength Training for Physical Education*. (Champaign, IL: Human Kinetics, 2025).

Power: Broad jump	Yes	Not yet
Swings the arms and pushes the hips back before takeoff		
Swings the arms forward, attempting to jump through the front wall		
Lands slowly, softly, and quietly, like a car coming to a stop sign		
Jumps from and lands on both feet equally		

From N. VanKouwenberg, *Functional Strength Training for Physical Education*. (Champaign, IL: Human Kinetics, 2025).

Power: Hang clean pull or hang high pull	Yes	Not yet
Stands with soft knees and the hands outside the legs; curls the knuckles under the bar		
Pulls the bar into the legs; scrapes the thigh with the bar until it hits the top of the knee		
Drives the top of the head through the ceiling, like jumping with the toes stuck		
Hang clean pull: arms stay locked; hang high pull: pulls the bar to the shirt collar with the knuckles down		

From N. VanKouwenberg, *Functional Strength Training for Physical Education*. (Champaign, IL: Human Kinetics, 2025).

Power: Hang power clean	Yes	Not Yet
Stands with soft knees and the hands outside the legs; curls the knuckles under the bar		
Pulls the bar into the legs and scrapes the thighs with the bar until it hits the tops of the knees		
Drives the top of the head through the ceiling, like jumping with the toes stuck		
Pulls the bar to the shirt collar; drops under the bar with the hips back and the elbows up		

From N. VanKouwenberg, *Functional Strength Training for Physical Education*. (Champaign, IL: Human Kinetics, 2025).

Core Exercise Checklists

Core: Plank	Yes	Not yet
Balances on the elbows and toes; the belly button is up, the tail is tucked, and the back is flat		
Makes a double chin		
The hands are flat; pulls the floor to the feet		
Braces as if in a hurricane		

From N. VanKouwenberg, *Functional Strength Training for Physical Education*. (Champaign, IL: Human Kinetics, 2025).

Core: Bird dog	Yes	Not yet
Makes a flat tabletop on the hands and knees		
Reaches with the opposite arm and leg		
Keeps the tabletop flat, like balancing a glass of water		
Returns to the starting position; repeats on the opposite side		

From N. VanKouwenberg, *Functional Strength Training for Physical Education*. (Champaign, IL: Human Kinetics, 2025).

Core: Staggered side plank	Yes	Not yet
Anchors the elbows into the ground, facing sideways		
The legs are separated like scissors, with the top leg forward		
Makes a double chin with the hips up and in, so the body is as straight as a board		
The opposite arm reaches to the sky, making a fist; braces as if in a hurricane		

From N. VanKouwenberg, *Functional Strength Training for Physical Education*. (Champaign, IL: Human Kinetics, 2025).

Core: Stability ball rollout	Yes	Not yet
Starts standing tall on the knees, with the arms locked and the hands together on top of the ball		
Slowly falls forward, rolling the ball under the arms		
Pulls the body back to the starting position		
Keeps the tail tucked and the back as straight as a board throughout		

From N. VanKouwenberg, *Functional Strength Training for Physical Education*. (Champaign, IL: Human Kinetics, 2025).

Sample Functional Movement Preparation

There are countless ways to design a quality comprehensive functional movement preparation to perform prior to a functional strength training workout. Regardless of the exercises selected, the objectives should be to

- increase the heart rate,
- increase blood flow,
- lubricate the joints,
- stretch major muscle groups,
- perform movements through a full range of motion,
- activate muscles to improve performance and decrease the risk of injury, and
- "wake up" the neuromuscular system.

Traditionally, exercises should be organized in a fashion that progresses from slow to fast and ground-based to locomotive. The following form is an example of a comprehensive functional movement preparation. You will find this form, along with video demonstrations of these exercises, in HK*Propel*.

Functional Movement Preparation

Soft-Tissue Quality

Full-body foam roll (5 min)

Static Stretch, Mobility, Activation, and Prehabilitation

Arm slides on back with roller squeeze between knees (10×)
Hamstring floss on back with ankle roll (5× on each leg)
One-leg hip lift with 3-sec hold (3× on each leg)
90-90 hip-mobility rocks (5× on each side)
90-90 hip rotations (5× on each side)
Double adductor stretch with T-spine rotations (5× on each side)
Ankle sit with shoulder rotations (5× in each direction)
Spiderman with rotation plus one-leg downward dog (3× each)
Toe touch to squat (5×)

Dynamic Stretch and Warm-Up

Standing quadriceps stretch with single leg Romanian deadlift to leg cradle and lunge (10 yd [9 m])
Alternating lateral squat to toe touch (10 yd [9 m])
High knees, butt kicks (10 yd [9 m] on each side)
Lateral skips (10 yd [9 m] on each side)
Carioca (10 yd [9 m] on each side)
Broad jump (3×)
Lateral leap with one-leg landing, then reset (3× on each side)
Submaximal backpedal or sprint starts (10-15 yd [9-14 m], 2-4×)

From N. VanKouwenberg, *Functional Strength Training for Physical Education*. (Champaign, IL: Human Kinetics, 2025).

Sample Functional Strength Training and High School Sport Performance Programs

This section provides examples of the middle and high school strength training workout routines discussed in chapter 10. Visit HK*Propel* for blank templates.

Middle School PE Functional Strength Training Workout Example

DAY 1			DAY 2		
Exercise	Sets	Repetitions or duration	Exercise	Sets	Repetitions
A1) Box jump	3	5	A1) Broad jump	3	3
A2) Goblet squat	3	5	A2) KB or hex deadlift	3	5
A3) TRX row	3	10	A3) Push-up	3	5-10
SUPERSET			SUPERSET		
B1) KB or hex deadlift	3	5	B1) Goblet squat	3	5
B2) Half-kneeling press	3	5 each	B2) TK pull-down	3	10
B3) Plank	3	20 sec	B3) Bird dog	3	5 each

Abbreviation: KB = kettlebell. TK= tall kneeling.

From N. VanKouwenberg, *Functional Strength Training for Physical Education*. (Champaign, IL: Human Kinetics, 2025).

High School PE Functional Strength Training Workout Example

DAY 1			DAY 2		
Exercise	Sets	Repetitions	Exercise	Sets	Repetitions or duration
A1) Broad jump	3	3	A1) Hang clean pull	3	5
A2) Front squat	3	5	A2) Split squat	3	5 each
A3) 1-Arm row	3	10 each	A3) Chin-up	3	5
SUPERSET			SUPERSET		
B1) BB bench press	3	5	B1) Hex deadlift	3	5
B2) Single leg RDL	3	5 each	B2) Half-kneeling press	3	5 each
B3) Stability ball rollout	3	8	B3) Stagger side plank	3	15 sec each

Abbreviations: BB = barbell; RDL = Romanian deadlift.

From N. VanKouwenberg, *Functional Strength Training for Physical Education*. (Champaign, IL: Human Kinetics, 2025).

High School Sport Performance Off-Season Program Example

Phase 1: Hypertrophy

DAY 1 MOVEMENT PREPARATION			DAY 2 MOVEMENT PREPARATION		
Exercise	Sets	Repetitions, distance, or duration	Exercise	Sets	Repetitions or duration
Box jump	3	5	Lateral leap, landing on both feet	3	3
Tall kneeling MB chest pass	3	5	MB scoop toss	3	4 each
Linear hurdle hop with pause	3	5 each	Agility ladder	3	2
Timed sprint	4	10 yd (9 m)	5-10-5 Pro agility	2	2
SUPERSET			SUPERSET		
RDL (2 wk eccentric, 2 wk isometric)	3	5 sec × 3	Hang clean pull	3	5
Broad jump	3	3	TK band pull apart	3	10
SUPERSET			SUPERSET		
Split squat	3	8 each	Front squat (2 wk eccentric, 2 wk isometric)	3	5 sec × 3
TK straight arm pulldown	3	10	Half-kneeling KB press	3	8
SUPERSET			SUPERSET		
Bench press (2 wk eccentric, 2 wk isometric)	3	5 sec × 3	Chin-up (2 wk eccentric, 2 wk isometric)	3	5 sec × 3
TRX row	3	10	Slideboard leg curl	3	8
Staggered side plank	3	15 sec each	Stability ball rollout	3	8

Abbreviations: KB = kettlebell; MB = medicine ball; TK = tall kneeling.

From N. VanKouwenberg, *Functional Strength Training for Physical Education*. (Champaign, IL: Human Kinetics, 2025).

Phase 2: Strength

DAY 1 MOVEMENT PREPARATION			DAY 2 MOVEMENT PREPARATION		
Exercise	Sets	Repetitions, distance, or duration	Exercise	Sets	Repetitions or duration
Tall hurdle jump with pause	3	4	Lateral leap, landing on both feet	3	3
Standing MB chest pass	3	5	MB scoop toss with step	3	4 each
Linear hurdle hop with double bounce	3	5 each	Agility ladder	3	2
Timed sprint	4	20 yd (18 m)	Change-of-direction races	4	7-10 sec
SUPERSET			SUPERSET		
RFESS	4	5 each	Hang power clean	4	4
Split jump	4	3 each	Half-kneeling shoulder CARs	3	5 each
SUPERSET			SUPERSET		
Hex deadlift	4	5	Goblet lateral squat	4	5 each
Half-kneeling face-pull	3	10	Standing landmine press	4	5 each
SUPERSET			SUPERSET		
DB bench press	4	5	Neutral grip chin-up	4	5
Standing 1-arm row	4	6 each	Single-leg RDL	4	5 each
Half-kneeling diagonal lift	3	8 each	Ab wheel rollout	3	8

Abbreviations: CAR = controlled articular rotation; DB = dumbbell; MB = medicine ball; RDL = Romanian deadlift; RFESS = rear foot elevated split squat.

From N. VanKouwenberg, *Functional Strength Training for Physical Education*. (Champaign, IL: Human Kinetics, 2025).

Phase 3: Maximum Strength and Power

DAY 1 MOVEMENT PREPARATION			DAY 2 MOVEMENT PREPARATION		
Exercise	Sets	Repetitions or distance	Exercise	Sets	Repetitions or duration
12 in. (30 cm) depth drop to broad jump	3	5	45-degree bounding	3	4 each
Sprint-start MB punch	3	3 each	MB scoop toss with shuffle	3	3 each
Linear hurdle hop with rebounding	3	5 each	Rebounding lateral and medial hurdle hop	3	4 each
Timed sprint	4	30 yd (27 m)	Reactive change-of-direction competition	4	7-10 sec
SUPERSET			SUPERSET		
Hex jump with pause (50%-75% body weight)	4	4	Hang power clean	4	3
TRX face-pull	3	8	Quadruped hip CARs	3	5 each
SUPERSET			SUPERSET		
Landmine push-press	4	4 each	Dynamic BB bench press	4	4
DB back elevated 1-leg hip lift	3	5 each	Single-leg RDL	3	4 each
SUPERSET			SUPERSET		
Single-leg squat	4	3 each	Pull-up	4	4
Kickstand 1-arm row	4	5 each	Goblet lateral lunge	4	4 each
Suitcase carry	3	30 yd (27 m) each	Body saw	3	8

Abbreviations: BB = barbell; CAR = controlled articular rotation; MB = medicine ball; RDL = Romanian deadlift; RFESS = rear foot elevated split squat.

From N. VanKouwenberg, *Functional Strength Training for Physical Education*. (Champaign, IL: Human Kinetics, 2025).

High School Sport Performance In-Season Program Example

DAY 1 MOVEMENT PREPARATION			DAY 2 MOVEMENT PREPARATION		
Exercise	Sets	Repetitions	Exercise	Sets	Repetitions
Split squat	4	3 each	Hex deadlift	4	3
TRX row	3	8	Tall kneeling band pull apart	3	10
SUPERSET			SUPERSET		
Single-leg RDL	3	4 each	DB bench press	3	5
Landmine press	3	5 each	Goblet lateral squat	3	4 each
SUPERSET			SUPERSET		
Chin-up	3	5	Standing 1-arm row	3	6 each
Stability ball rollout	3	8	Staggered side plank	3	:15 each

Abbreviations: DB = dumbbell; RDL = Romanian deadlift.

From N. VanKouwenberg, *Functional Strength Training for Physical Education*. (Champaign, IL: Human Kinetics, 2025).

Bibliography

Baechle, T.R., and R.W. Earle. 2008. *Essentials of Strength Training and Conditioning.* 3rd ed. Champaign, IL: Human Kinetics.

Balyi, I., R. Way, and C. Higgs. 2013. *Long-Term Athlete Development.* Champaign, IL: Human Kinetics.

Bartholomew, B. 2023. "Coaching Cues - Science for Sport." Scienceforsport.com. May 30, 2023. https://www.scienceforsport.com/coaching-cues/#toggle-id-1.

Behm, D., and J.C. Colado. 2012. "The Effectiveness of Resistance Training Using Unstable Surfaces and Devices for Rehabilitation." *International Journal of Sports Physical Therapy* 7: 226-41. www.ncbi.nlm.nih.gov/pmc/articles/PMC3325639.

Boyle, M. 2016. *New Functional Training for Sports.* Champaign, IL: Human Kinetics.

Boyle, M. 2023. *Designing Strength Training Programs and Facilities.* 2nd ed. Aptos, CA: On Target Publications.

Dahab, K.S., and T.M. McCambridge. 2009. "Strength Training in Children and Adolescents: Raising the Bar for Young Athletes?" *Sports Health: A Multidisciplinary Approach* 1 (3): 226. https://doi.org/10.1177/1941738109334215.

David, D., C. Giannini, F. Chiarelli, and A. Mohn. 2021. "Text Neck Syndrome in Children and Adolescents." *International Journal of Environmental Research and Public Health* 18 (4): 1565. www.mdpi.com/1660-4601/18/4/1565/htm.

Davidson, K. 2021. "Does Fat Turn into Muscle? What to Know." *Healthline*, March 2, 2021. www.healthline.com/nutrition/does-fat-turn-into-muscle.

Dechant, Z. 2018. *Movement Over Maxes: Developing the Foundation for Baseball Performance.* Self-published, Zach Dechant.

Dietz, Z., and B. Peterson. 2012. *Triphasic Training: A Systematic Approach to Elite Speed and Explosive Strength Performance.* Hudson, WI: Bye Dietz Sport Enterprise.

Donskov, A. 2016. *Physical Preparation for Ice Hockey.* Bloomington, IN: AuthorHouse.

Donskov, A. 2020. *The Gain, Go, Grow Manual: Programming for High Performance Hockey Players.* Bloomington, IN: AuthorHouse.

Feito, Y., E.K. Burrows, and L.P. Tabb. 2018. "A 4-Year Analysis of the Incidence of Injuries Among CrossFit-Trained Participants." *Orthopedic Journal of Sports Medicine* 6 (10): 2325967118803100. https://doi.org/10.1177/2325967118803100.

Gordon, B.R., C.P. McDowell, M. Lyons, and M.P. Herring. 2020. "Resistance Exercise Training for Anxiety and Worry Symptoms Among Young Adults: A Randomized Controlled Trial." *Scientific Reports* 10 (1): 17548. https://doi.org/10.1038/s41598-020-74608-6.

Gustavo, S.Z., S.S. Pinto, M.R. Silva, D.B. Dolinski, and C.L. Alberton. 2018. "Whole-Body High-Intensity Interval Training Induce Similar Cardiorespiratory Adaptations Compared With Traditional High-Intensity Interval Training and Moderate-Intensity Continuous Training in Healthy Men." *Journal of Strength and Conditioning Research* 32 (10): 2730-42. https://pubmed.ncbi.nlm.nih.gov/29746386.

Handelsman, D.J., A.L. Hirschberg, and S. Bermon. 2018. "Circulating Testosterone as the Hormonal Basis of Sex Differences in Athletic Performance." *Endocrine Reviews* 39 (5): 803-29. https://doi.org/10.1210/er.2018-00020.

Hill, J.O., H.R. Wyatt, and J.C. Peters. 2012. "Energy Balance and Obesity." *Circulation* 126 (1): 126-32. www.ncbi.nlm.nih.gov/pmc/articles/PMC3401553.

Karimian, R., N. Rahnama, G. Ghasemi, and S. Lenjannejadian. 2019. "Photogrammetric Analysis of Upper Cross Syndrome Among Teachers and the Effects of National Academy of Sports Medicine Exercises With Ergonomic Intervention on the Syndrome." *Journal of Research in Health Sciences* 19 (3): e00450. www.ncbi.nlm.nih.gov/pmc/articles/PMC7183553.

Lauersen, J.B., D.M. Bertelsen, and L.B. Andersen. 2013. "The Effectiveness of Exercise Interventions to Prevent Sports Injuries: A Systematic Review and Meta-Analysis of Randomized Controlled Trials." *British Journal of Sports Medicine* 48 (11): 871-77. https://doi.org/10.1136/bjsports-2013-092538.

Leite, T.B., P.B. Costa, R.D. Leite, J.S. Novaes, S.J. Fleck, and R. Simão. 2017. "Effects of Different Number of Sets of Resistance Training on Flexibility." *International Journal of Exercise Science* 10 (3): 354-64. www.ncbi.nlm.nih.gov/pmc/articles/PMC5609666.

Leong, D.P., K.K. Teo., S. Rangarajan, P. Lopez-Jaramillo, A. Avezum, A. Orlandini, P. Seron, et al. 2015. "Prognostic Value of Grip Strength: Findings From the Prospective Urban Rural Epidemiology (PURE) Study." *The Lancet* 386 (9990): 266-73. https://doi.org/10.1016/s0140-6736(14)62000-6.

LeWine, H. 2015. "Grip Strength May Provide Clues to Heart Health." *Harvard Health Blog*, May 19, 2015. www.health.harvard.edu/blog/grip-strength-may-provide-clues-to-heart-health-201505198022.

National Heart, Lung, and Blood Institute . 2019. "Calculate Your BMI - Standard BMI Calculator." Nih.gov. U.S. Department of Health & Human Services. 2019. https://www.nhlbi.nih.gov/health/educational/lose_wt/BMI/bmicalc.htm.

Rearick, B. 2020. *Coaching Rules: A How-to Manual for a Successful Career in Strength and Fitness*. Aptos, CA: On Target Publications.

Schoenfeld, B.J., J. Grgic, D.W. Van Every, and D.L. Plotkin. 2021. "Loading Recommendations for Muscle Strength, Hypertrophy, and Local Endurance: A Re-Examination of the Repetition Continuum." *Sports* 9 (2): 32. https://doi.org/10.3390/sports9020032.

Seitz, L.B., A.A. Reyes, T.T. Tran, E. Saez de Villarreal, and G.G. Haff. 2014. "Increases in Lower-Body Strength Transfer Positively to Sprint Performance: A Systematic Review With Meta-Analysis." Sports Medicine 44 (12): 1693-702. https://pubmed.ncbi.nlm.nih.gov/25059334.

Sharma, A., V. Madaan, and F.D. Petty. 2006. "Exercise for Mental Health." *Primary Care Companion to the Journal of Clinical Psychiatry* 8 (2): 106. www.ncbi.nlm.nih.gov/pmc/articles/PMC1470658.

Stenger, L. 2018. "What Is Functional/Neuromotor Fitness?" *ACSM'S Health & Fitness Journal* 22 (6): 35-43. https://doi.org/10.1249/fit.0000000000000439.

Teraoka, E., H.J. Ferreira, D. Kirk, and F. Bardid. 2020. "Affective Learning in Physical Education: A Systematic Review." *Journal of Teaching in Physical Education* 40 (3): 460-473. https://doi.org/10.1123/jtpe.2019-0164.

Unify Health Team. 2021. "What Are the Five Components of Fitness?" Unify Health Labs. March 17, 2021. www.unifyhealthlabs.com/what-are-the-five-components-of-fitness.

U.S. National Library of Medicine. 2020. "Patellofemoral Pain Syndrome (Runner's Knee): Overview." Last modified August 13, 2020. www.ncbi.nlm.nih.gov/books/NBK561507.

Westcott, W.L. 2012. "Resistance Training Is Medicine: Effects of Strength Training on Health." *Current Sports Medicine Reports* 11 (4): 209-16. https://pubmed.ncbi.nlm.nih.gov/22777332.

Winkelman, N. 2020. *The Language of Coaching: The Art & Science of Teaching Movement.* Champaign, IL: Human Kinetics.

Xiao, W., K.G. Soh, M.R. Wazir, O. Talib, X. Bai, T. Bu, H. Sun, et al. 2021. "Effect of Functional Training on Physical Fitness Among Athletes: A Systematic Review." *Frontiers in Physiology* 12: 738878. https://doi.org/10.3389/fphys.2021.738878.

About the Author

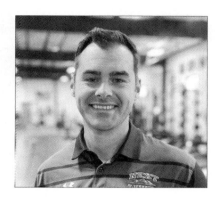

Nate VanKouwenberg, CFSC, is a physical education teacher and strength and conditioning coordinator in the Victor Central School District in New York. Using his experience developing Victor's K-12 functional strength training curriculum, VanKouwenberg has created a comprehensive professional development workshop for teachers, coaches, athletic directors, and college students called Functional Strength Training for PE. He has presented at countless conferences and school districts over the years to improve the quality of physical education fitness units and high school strength and conditioning programs.

In addition, VanKouwenberg is the founder and owner of Next Level Strength & Conditioning in Rochester, New York. Since 2004, Next Level has helped a wide range of athletes and general fitness enthusiasts reach their goals. Aside from his role on the business and staff development side of Next Level, he also coaches their Pro Total Hockey Training group each summer. He served as the strength and conditioning coach for the Rochester Institute of Technology (RIT) Division I men's hockey team for eight seasons.

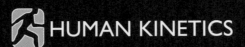

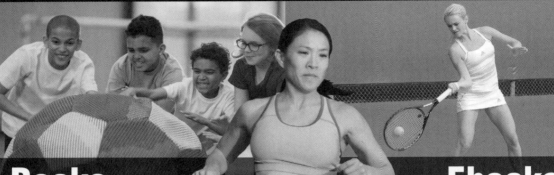

Books   **Ebooks**

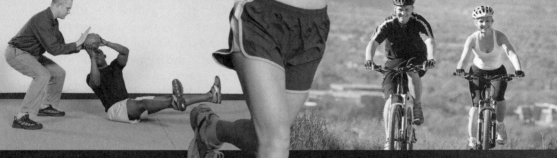

Continuing Education   **Journals ...and more!**

US.HumanKinetics.com
Canada.HumanKinetics.com

Sign up for our newsletters!
Get the latest insights with regular newsletters, plus periodic product information and special insider offers from Human Kinetics.